that Fit Life

How to transform
your life,
lose weight,
and keep it off!

JEREMY B. GOODMAN

Inspired Vision
PUBLISHING

That Fit Life: How to transform your life, lose weight, and keep it off!

For information regarding special discounts for bulk purchases, please send email to sales@inspiredvisionpublishing.com.

Paperback ISBN: 978-1-7378852-0-7
Hardcover ISBN: 978-1-7378852-2-1

Book Cover Design by Rodjie Ulanday

Printed in USA

Inspired Vision
PUBLISHING

Dedication

I dedicate this book to my wife Lakisha
and my daughters Teairra and Lakeya.
I thank God every day
for blessing me with his angels.

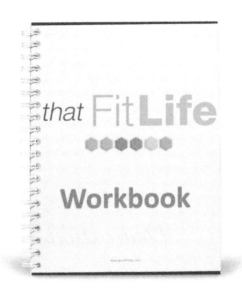

DOWNLOAD THE WORKBOOK

Just to say thanks for buying my book, I would like to give you the Workbook 100% FREE!

TO DOWNLOAD GO TO:
https://jgoodfitness.com/that-fit-life

Contents

Introduction

I'm on a mission to help as many people as I can to overcome their weight-loss struggles and reach their health and fitness goals. I have a deep passion for helping people, and I feel that my knowledge can make a difference.

This book is a culmination of personal experience, education, self-study, research, and experimentation. I've learned so much from my journey, and I hope this book will serve as a guide to help others accomplish their goals and achieve their dream bodies. The information in this book will help transform you mentally, physically, and spiritually.

This book is for people who are looking for a realistic approach to reaching their health and fitness goals. No fads, no gimmicks—nothing but effective and proven principles designed to transform your life. This book is for the person who is struggling to achieve his/her ideal weight. This book is for the person who knows what to do but needs help with structure and compliance.

This book will help so many people regardless of their health and fitness goals because it is a book on how to live a lifestyle where health and fitness are top priorities. I call that kind of life, *That Fit Life*. It's the life I've been living for over twenty years.

My journey began in the fall of 1999. This was my senior year of high school, and my weight topped out at 307 pounds. My mother was extremely concerned about my health. She had me go to the doctor because she was concerned about my weight and how loud I was snoring at night.

The doctor evaluated me and explained that by definition, I was obese. I had to lose weight or I would be at high risk for serious health issues like diabetes, high blood pressure, high cholesterol, etc.

The doctor referred me to a dietitian, who provided me with some basic nutritional information and helped me set a goal. My original goal was to get down to 200 pounds; my dream goal was to get to 170 pounds.

I was fascinated by the information I received about nutrition and exercise. This was my first exposure to the importance of calories, macronutrients, weight management, exercising regularly, and staying active.

With this advice from my family doctor and dietician, I changed my diet and started exercising at home. By the end of my senior year, I had lost almost seventy pounds. I felt amazing. The following fall, I entered college as a new man. A lighter man.

In the first year of college, I was still overweight, but I was in far better condition compared to my heaviest weight in 1999. I maintained my weight well. In the summer of 2001, I went home for summer break, and by the end of the summer, I was down to 190 pounds. I had passed my goal of 200 pounds! I felt so good going into my sophomore year in college, having met my original goal. Now my heart was set on reaching my dream goal of 170 pounds.

From the summer of 2001 to the summer of 2014, my weight fluctuated from 190 pounds to 230 pounds. For exactly one week in 2009, I dropped below 180 pounds, but it was very short-lived and I did not see those types of numbers again for many years. During this time period, I went on countless weight-loss campaigns, tried every type of diet, tried every type of gym routine, watched hundreds of exercise videos, and read many books. Nothing seemed to stick. Every year, I repeated the same old New Year's resolution to lose weight and reach that 170-pound goal.

In January 2014, I was around 230 pounds. My wife's cousin was getting married in the summer, and I set a goal to get in shape for the wedding. I was very determined. By March of that year, I had lost a few pounds and was on the right track.

At the time, my only exercise was running. No weights, no other types of exercise—just running. I ended up injuring my foot and was sidelined for several weeks. Since I wasn't engaged in any other form of exercise, I did nothing and slowly slid back into my poor nutrition habits. By the time the summer wedding rolled around, I was a whopping 250 pounds. This was the heaviest I'd been since my high school days. I was so disappointed in myself.

This moment was a major turning point in my life. I made a promise to myself that I would do everything in my power to lose weight and gain control of my life. I had to release myself from past mistakes and adopt a healthier lifestyle. I had to make health and fitness my top priorities.

Over the next year, I worked hard to transform my life and became a better version of myself. I went from being obese and squishy to lean and fit. I went from 250 pounds to 170 pounds. I finally met my goal! Not only did I lose weight, but my entire life changed.

Easier said than done, right? You are probably wondering, "Okay, but what did you do? How did you finally reach your goal?"

This book reveals all the key lessons and principles I used to transform myself mentally, physically, and spiritually. I will teach you my blueprint to losing weight and keeping it off for good, also known as the **Fit Life Pillars**. This book will remove all the guesswork and focus on the important things to help you transform your life.

Essentially, I'm going to show you how to live *That Fit Life*.

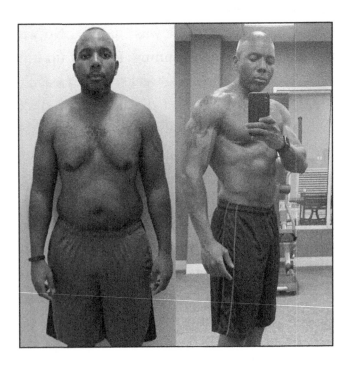

I've been where you are. I empathize with those who are struggling to lose weight. I understand what it's like to be severely overweight. I understand the challenges that come with comfort eating and stress eating. I understand how being overweight can lead to depression and anxiety. I understand the challenges people face when they are on an endless weight-loss journey.

My vision is to live a healthy and active lifestyle that inspires others to do the same. I have a passion for helping people become the best versions of themselves by losing weight and keeping it off. My mission is to transform lives.

So let's get started!

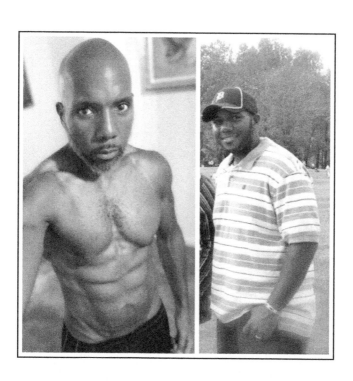

The Fit Life Pillars

Health and fitness are a lifelong journey. I often refer to this journey as *That Fit Life*. Living *That Fit Life* enhances your quality of life into a life of continuous improvement and learning. I would like to introduce you to the blueprint for living *That Fit Life:* The Fit Life Pillars! There are six pillars that make up the Fit Life Pillars: Mental, Nutrition, Physical, Social, Spiritual, and Essential.

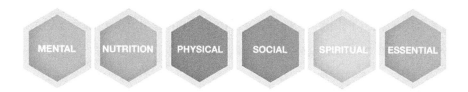

While I have a chapter dedicated to each of the six Fit Life Pillars, let's go over a brief description of the Pillars before diving deeper:

Mental Pillar

The Mental Pillar focuses on training your mind for success and adopting the right mindset to help you accomplish your goals.

This pillar is so important because it defines what's important to you and how you will take action.

Nutrition Pillar

The Nutrition Pillar focuses on how to design the best nutrition approach that works best for you. With nutrition, it's never a one-size-fits-all.

Physical Pillar

The Physical Pillar breaks down all the key things you need to know about weight training and cardio. Yes, both! Weight training and cardio are *both* key for weight loss and for maintenance.

Social Pillar

The Social Pillar highlights key areas where you can reach out to others for support to help you along your journey.

Spiritual Pillar

The Spiritual Pillar takes a deep look inside and focuses on how we can tap into the greatness inside of us.

Essential Pillar

The Essential Pillar highlights additional areas that will accelerate your progress and help you achieve your weight-loss goals.

The Pillars are the guiding principles that will help you take back your life and get you out of the vicious weight-loss cycle. The Pillars will help you transform mentally, physically, and spiritually, and they will set you on a path toward living an active & healthy lifestyle!

Chapter 1
Mental Pillar

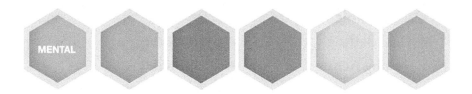

"Discipline is the bridge between goals and accomplishment."

- Jim Rohn

Chapter 1 Introduction

Weight-loss success begins with the mind. No nutrition or exercise plan stands a chance of being sustainable without the right mindset. The Mental Pillar is the most important because it provides you with a strong foundation. It focuses on training your mind for success and adopting the right mindset to help you accomplish your goals. This also defines what's important to you and lays out how you will take action toward achievement. In this chapter, we are going to explore the following topics:

• Know Your Why	• Eliminating Distractions
• Commitment	• 5 Ds
• Goal Setting	• Motivation
• Taking Action	• Consistency
• Mindset	• Self-Awareness
• Vision Board	• Mastery of Self
• Habits	• Self-Control
• Positive Self-Talk	• Dream
• Affirmations	• Believe in Yourself

The wisdom I've gained from the Mental Pillar was powerful and life-changing. For many years, I struggled with my weight. It seemed like I tried everything under the sun. I was trying so many tactics to lose weight, but none of them worked because I did not truly know myself or what was best for me. I had to get my mind right. I had to learn how to train my mind for success.

This chapter will highlight powerful and life-changing ways you can train your mind for success to build a strong foundation for future growth.

Know Your Why

Before starting this fit-life journey, it's important to understand your "Why"—in other words, your purpose or reason for starting this journey. *Why* do you want to pursue your goal? *Why* is this goal important to you?

Usually, the answers to these questions are personal and have specific meanings. Depending on the stage you are at in your life, your "why" may be your greatest source of motivation and inspiration.

Over the years, I've learned it's not enough to know what you are doing or how you are doing it. A deeper and more impactful source of motivation is knowing why you are doing it. I encourage you to give this some serious thought and take time right now to write out your why and uncover your deepest desires.

This list will serve as your motivation and keep you moving toward your goals. I performed this exercise at the beginning of my transformation. This was a critical step in the journey because it uncovered my wants and desires. This will serve as a useful tool in your journey. Your list may look much different, but I will share my list to give you a good example:

<u>My Why:</u>

- I want to live an active and healthy lifestyle
- I want to be a positive role model and live by example
- I want to be able to keep up with my active kids
- I want to look sexy for my wife
- Reaching my goal will open the doors to higher career and personal achievement

- I want to be at a healthy weight
- I want to have a healthy body-fat percentage
- I want to have a healthy Body Mass Index (BMI) (25 or less)
- I want to be able to run races: marathons, half-marathons, 5ks, etc.
- I want to increase my self-confidence
- I want to increase my self-esteem
- I want to wear size 32 inch or smaller pants
- I want to wear large- or medium-size shirts
- I want to be more energetic
- I want to pull my shirt off in public and not be embarrassed
- I want to look and feel younger

This exercise revealed way more about my reason for living *That Fit Life* than me just wanting to lose weight. As you can see, it went much deeper than that. Whenever I need some motivation or need to reset my thinking, I pull out my list and read it several times. After reading my list, I often get emotionally charged and ready to get rolling again.

One of my favorite quotes is from German philosopher Frederick Nietzsche. He once wrote, "He who has a why to live for can bear almost any how." Knowing your why is a key step in figuring out how to achieve the goals that are important to you.

Always ask yourself, "Why?" Whenever you face a major decision or are struggling to prioritize your goals, ask yourself, "Why is this important to me?"

Action Steps

✓ Make a list of your whys.

✓ Save your list and place it in a location where you can easily retrieve it for future reference. I wrote mine in a journal and have an electronic version of the list stored in the Notes app on my phone.

Commitment

Have you ever tried losing weight, gaining lean muscle, or improving your endurance—and failed? It's discouraging and depressing when you put in so much work and effort, yet cannot reach your goal. I've been down this road. The main reason I failed to reach my goals in the past was that I didn't commit to them. Sure, I may have thought about my goals and may have taken some action, but I did not fully commit to reaching them.

I thought long and hard about my failed attempts, and I found a pattern: I did not make a genuine commitment.

If you are serious about reaching your goals, you have to make a commitment to do so. When you make a commitment, you are basically making a promise to follow through. This type of promise is powerful because it is a promise to yourself *and* a promise to the people you care most about.

Look at your list of "reasons why" that you created in the previous section. I bet your reasons are both for yourself and for the people you care most about. When you make a commitment for yourself and those you care about, you have a greater chance of following through to the end. You don't have to worry about failing when you commit to reaching your goals.

The commitment you are making is also a promise that you are willing to make changes and do what it takes to accomplish your goals. Getting from where you are now to where you want to be will require change and action. In addition, it will require you to stay the course despite the challenges you will inevitably face. Making a commitment to a goal or dream is one of the fundamental principles of success.

In the summer of 2014, I made a commitment to reach my goal weight, and I shared that commitment with my wife, my children, my family members, and my friends to gain their support. When you commit to your goals and share your goals with those you care most about, you will be more successful in reaching your goals. Plus, you will strengthen your relationships. This one revelation, this one simple, powerful action set me up for a life-changing transformation.

Commitments influence your thoughts and actions. For example, after making my commitment to reach my goal weight, I joined the local gym. This put me in an atmosphere that supported my goals and surrounded me with people who shared common interests. I developed new friendships, began reading health and fitness articles, signed up for various newsletters, and followed blogs. The information I was consuming changed my thoughts. As this process continued to unfold, it guided me toward achieving my goal.

Accomplishing any worthwhile goal takes time, effort, and commitment. A serious commitment will require full investment in your goal. It's more than just spoken words or sentences on a page. To stay committed to your goal, you need to set SMART goals and have the right mindset, which we will cover in the next section.

Are you committed to your goals or dreams? If not, this is the time to get serious.

Action Steps

✓ Make a promise to yourself and to those you care about that you are willing to make changes and do what it takes to accomplish your goals.

✓ Put your commitment down in writing and share it with the people you care about.

✓ Take action and focus on the things that will drive you closer to your goals.

Goal Setting

Goal setting is a powerful process for determining the type of future you want to create and bringing your dreams into reality. Stephen R. Covey said it best in his popular book, *The 7 Habits of Highly Effective People*: "Begin with the end in mind."[1]

Goal setting is an extremely important step when trying to achieve any type of success in life. Goals provide direction and help guide your actions. Written goals are the vehicles that bring your dreams into reality.

If you want to lose weight and keep it off, you need to have well-defined goals. First, consider what you want to achieve, and then write your goals down to make them tangible. Next, you want to make your goals SMART. SMART is an acronym that has several variations floating around. The one I like to use breaks it down as follows:

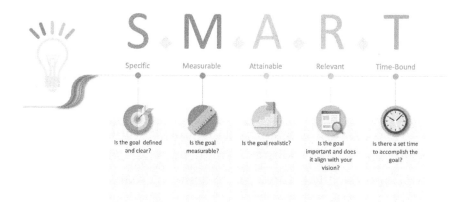

- **Specific** - Your goal should be clear and specific. If your goal is too general, you will not get the desired outcome.

- **Measurable** - Your goal needs to be specific enough for you to measure and track your progress. If you can't measure your goal, how do you know if you are on the right track?
- **Attainable** - Your goal needs to be realistic and attainable. If you set a goal that cannot be achieved, you are going to face a great deal of disappointment.
- **Relevant** - Your goal needs to be relevant to you and what you want. Does your goal align with your vision or desired outcome? Is this the right goal for you currently?
- **Time Bound** - To drive the right behaviors and actions, your goals need to have a target date. This will help you prioritize your actions and allow you to focus on your goals.

SMART goals allow you to set powerful goals rather than generic goals. For example, setting a goal to "lose weight" sounds good and all, but it is not clear or specific enough. How much weight do you want to lose, and what time frame do you want to lose it by? General, non-specific goals do not provide any direction or specific target for you to achieve.

Using the SMART approach, a good example of a goal would be: "I want to lose five pounds by December 30th, in time for my 10-year anniversary." This example meets the requirements of a SMART goal: the goal is specific, measurable, achievable, relevant, and is time-bound. Structuring your goals using the SMART approach will allow you to achieve great success.

Below are additional examples of SMART goals:

General, non-specific goal	SMART goal
I am going to eat more protein	I am going to eat three meals per day that contain at least 20 grams of protein for the next three weeks
I am going to lift weights	I am going to perform a full-body weight-training routine on Monday, Wednesday, and Friday at 5:30 am in my basement for the next six weeks.
I am going to drink more water	I will drink 64-128 ounces of water every weekday until December 15th
I am going to start running every week.	I will run for 30 minutes three times a week for six weeks starting Monday, July 1st

When setting goals, it is important to set long-term and short-term goals. The best approach is to break your goals down into manageable time frames:

- Yearly
- Monthly
- Weekly
- Daily

This approach will provide you with the most direction and stimulate the right action at the right time.

Once you determine your goals and make them SMART, you need to post them in places that are highly visible and review them daily. This will keep your goals in front of you and at the top of your priority list. I like to think of it as your own personal advertising. In this case, you get to choose the advertising you are exposed to and view it as much as you like. I like to write my goals out on several index cards and post them in various locations in my home, office, car, and in my wallet. A good spot to post your goals is on a vision board, which we will cover soon.

It's time to take some action!

Action Steps

✓ Determine what you want to achieve and write out your goals. Make sure your goals are SMART.

✓ Post your goals in highly visible areas and keep a copy on you for reference.

✓ Review your goals daily until you accomplish them.

✓ Once you achieve your goals, develop new SMART goals and repeat these steps.

Taking Action

Once you understand your why, have made your commitment, and set your SMART goals, it's time to start taking action toward accomplishing your weight-loss goals. This step is what separates those who are successful at weight loss and those who are not.

Don't get caught up in analysis paralysis or waiting for the perfect moment to start. Take action right away and start building momentum.

Taking the steps to lose weight can be challenging. There are so many factors that come into play, and it's important to not get overwhelmed with all the information and hype.

The key is to keep it simple and start with small daily actions. These daily actions will build momentum over time and help you reach your goals.

To ensure you are taking the right actions, be sure to focus on the behaviors and habits needed to achieve your desired goal or outcome. By focusing on the behaviors and habits, you will establish a strong foundation to build on. In addition, behaviors and habits are repeatable, and if you want to make consistent progress toward your goals, you need repeatable actions. For example, keeping the fridge stocked with healthy foods and meal prepping are repeatable actions that will help you with your weight-loss goals. Another repeatable action is picking out your gym clothes the night before and having your gym bag ready for your next workout. Repeating simple daily actions like these over a long period of time will build momentum and help you reach your goals.

You will not reach your goals if you are not taking action! You can't wish for it; you must work for it every day.

Relentless Pursuit of Goal

If you are serious about reaching your weight-loss goals, you need to be *relentless!* A relentless person is someone who keeps trying and never gives up. There are so many distractions that can derail you from reaching your goals. One way to battle these distractions and protect yourself from excuses is to always stay determined and persistent. For example, if you have one bad meal, don't give up and throw the whole day away. Focus on the next healthy meal and keep moving forward. Another good example, let's say the gym closed due to a power outage. Instead of skipping your workout, you can head home or go to the park to work out.

I want to take this time to talk about how relentless I was in pursuing my goal. I got to the point where I would not allow anyone or anything to get in the way of accomplishing my goal. While pursuing my health and fitness goals, I developed a new mental muscle of determination that translated into all areas of my life. Maybe it was always there, but I just didn't know how to develop or tap into it before. This muscle allows me to exercise extreme focus and quickly eliminate distractions. In other words, I am now able to get into the zone!

When you become relentless and decide that you are willing to do whatever it takes, you will reach your goals! If you fall seven times, get back up eight times and keep at it!

Reflection

Are you willing and ready to put in the work? Are you willing to give it your all? Are you going to let any obstacle get in your way? Are you going to let distractions derail you, or send you in the wrong direction?

Those are some tough questions. They are things you need to think about as you embark on your weight-loss journey.

Mindset

The key to getting in the best shape of your life—and having a successful life in general—is acquiring the right mindset. A person's ability to stick with an exercise or nutrition program can be related to their mindset, or their way of thinking. For example, if a person finds exercise and nutrition to be boring or difficult, the chances of them sticking with or even starting a program are slim. Compare this to a person who finds exercise and nutrition to be interesting, helpful, and even fun; they will have a far better chance of sticking with a program and achieving success.

Mindset played a key role in my transformation. I've tried some of the best exercise and nutrition programs in existence, but I did not see results because I had a failure mindset. This is a mindset where thinking is fixed, quits when situations begin to get challenging, and disregards small wins due to an all or nothing mentality. I spent many years starting and quitting because of this, and I was getting nowhere fast.

This experience taught me the importance of having the right mindset. When I provide coaching to my clients, I focus heavily on mindset and goal setting at the start. If we can get this part nailed down in the beginning, the exercise and nutrition become simple.

Here are five simple steps to get into the right mindset for your health and fitness journey:

1)   **Set SMART Goals** - In the previous section, I covered the importance of setting SMART goals and provided the action steps to take in order to launch you on the right path.

2) **Develop a "No Excuses" Mentality** - A "no excuses" mentality means you will not allow any excuses to stand in the way of reaching your goals.

3) **Mastery of Self** - You need to develop a high level of self-awareness and self-control. At times, we can be our own worst enemy. Learning to master your thoughts, emotions, and actions can lead to a healthier, more productive life. A book I highly recommend to help you develop a high sense of self-awareness and self-control is *Search Inside Yourself* written by Chad-Meng Tan. The book is based on the mindfulness-based emotional intelligence curriculum by the same name that started at Google in 2007[2]. It's one of my top five favorite books.

4) **Be Positive** - Positive thinking goes hand in hand with success. Positive thinking brings about optimism and will motivate you toward success. As mentioned above, a person with a positive view of exercise and nutrition has a better chance of sticking with a program.

5) **Have Fun** - Find a program and/or trainer that you enjoy working with. Successful people enjoy what they are doing and learn to have fun along the way!

Action Steps

✓ Reflect on your way of thinking. Do you have the right mindset to succeed, or is your success limited by doubt, excuses, and negativity? If so, follow the five steps to get you into the right mindset.

✓ If you have not developed your SMART Goals, please stop right now and develop your SMART Goals.

Vision Board

A vision board is a collage of images and/or words representing a person's dreams, desires, or goals. The main purpose of the vision board is to serve as a symbolic source of inspiration and motivation. Vision boards are meant to be personal and are super fun to make.

Below is a picture of my vision board in my house. It is filled with words, pictures, cutouts, magnets, documents, quotes, affirmations, and anything else that represents my big goals and dreams in life. My goal to write and publish this book was on my board.

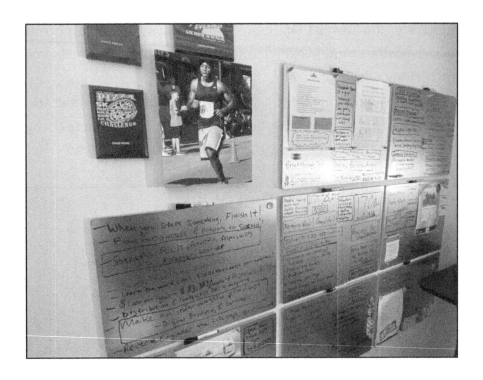

I have a large section on my vision board specifically for health and fitness. During my weight-loss transformation, I would review my vision board at least once a day. It helped me stay focused and inspired me to continue the journey until I reached my health and fitness goals.

One of the most motivating aspects of my vision board was a section where I kept track of my weight each week. I started tracking my weight when I was at 250 pounds, and once a week I would post the number on my board. It was awesome seeing my weight drop week by week; my big goal of getting down to 170 became more real as time went by. The day I wrote "170 pounds" on my board was one of the best days of my life.

Over time, I realized how powerful and life-changing vision boards are. Many of my major goals I've written on my board have been accomplished, and with more time and patience, the rest of my dreams and goals will be achieved, too.

There are many ways to go about creating a vision board—there are even several workshops and classes on creating vision boards. Below is a quick guide to get started on creating a vision board:

Materials Needed:

- Poster board, dry-erase board, cork board, or small canvas
- Magazine clippings, pictures, or other visuals that represent your goals
- Scissors, markers, paint, glue, tape, pins, or tacks

Step 1 - Take a few moments to reflect on your dreams and big goals

Step 2 - Grab your materials and begin creating your board

Step 3 - Begin posting the clippings, pictures, or other visuals that represent your dreams and big goals onto your board

Step 4 - Use your markers or paint to write in quotes, affirmations, and other words or phrases that inspire and motivate you to pursue your goal

Step 5 - Find a space in your home or office to display or hang your board. Place it in an easily accessible area where you'll see it every day

I encourage you to take the time to create a vision board that will motivate and inspire you every day. Many people and celebrities have used vision boards to help them visualize and help bring their dreams to reality. Personally, it was a game-changer.

Action Step

✓ After creating your vision board, I recommend taking a picture and saving it. This picture will serve as a back-up in the event items are removed from the board or information is erased inadvertently.

Habits

I often tell people I am a creature of habit. I'm big on having routines that help make my life more efficient, and my routines are a collection of my daily habits.

A habit is something that you do often or regularly. Habits can be either conscious or subconscious and are the driving factors behind how you behave daily. Our brains have the unique ability to take habits (good or bad) and put them on autopilot because, according to experts in science and in psychology, the brain is constantly looking for ways to be more efficient. For example, a team of researchers from the University of Southern California conducted field experiments using testing conditions under which people ate out of habit. They found that people ate out of habit regardless of motivational influences.[3]

It's extremely important to understand the habits that drive your daily behaviors. Habits can make you or break you when it comes to living a healthy lifestyle, as good habits take a while to form, and bad habits take a while to break.

Adopting healthy lifestyle habits will allow you to lose weight and keep it off. Healthy habits like eating fruits and veggies, drinking water, working out daily, getting quality sleep, and reviewing your daily goals are a few good examples.

Establishing a healthy lifestyle routine was a winning strategy during my journey. My routine was not some elaborate or complex system; it comprised simple habits and behaviors that I executed daily. This led me to develop a morning and evening routine that jump-started and ended my day on good notes.

My morning and evening routine

I'm a big believer in having a set morning and evening routine. This structured start and end of my day was an effective habit that supported my weight-loss journey.

The first thing I do in my supercharged morning routine is wake up every day at 4:00 a.m. When I wake up, I instantly jump out of bed to prevent myself from climbing back under the covers or hitting the snooze button. These precious seconds can be the difference between an awesome day or a mediocre one. The law of dynamics comes into play here: a body in motion stays in motion. Get up! Let's go!

After successfully jumping out of bed, I take a moment to thank God for blessing me with another day and read a Bible scripture. I reflect on how good he has been to me. I do this every morning without fail. I love starting my day by connecting and strengthening my relationship with God.

The next thing I do as a part of my morning routine is head into the kitchen to drink some water. Every morning, I drink two cups of water. Proper hydration is so essential (I cover hydration in more detail in Chapter 6); the body needs water after a full night's rest, as it loses a considerable amount of water during sleep. Your body uses water during sleep to repair, rejuvenate, and replenish the cells, as well as support other critical functions.

After I finish drinking my water every morning, I meditate for 20 minutes. I love starting my day with meditation. Meditation allows me to be more in tune with my mind and body (I cover meditation in more detail in Chapter 6). After I meditate, I get dressed and make my way to the gym for an awesome workout.

When I return from my workout, I prepare and enjoy a healthy breakfast.

My evening routine usually starts 45 minutes to an hour prior to going to bed. The first thing I do is make up my bed and fluff my pillows. This habit is extremely helpful, as it helps get my mind geared toward sleep and signals my brain to wind down. After getting my bed ready, I pick out and set aside my gym clothes for my morning workout. Next, I update my journal with my stats and notes for the day. After updating my journal, I review my vision board and read my goals and affirmations out loud. Finally, with the time I have left I turn off the TV and I read a book until bedtime. I repeat this process every night, without skipping a beat.

This has become my set routine over time. Now, I execute it daily with little thought or effort. This routine helped me in my weight-loss journey and this same routine is helping me keep the weight off today. I encourage you to find a morning and/ or evening routine that works for you and that will help you structure your day to maximize your potential.

Consistency

Consistency is so important for losing weight and keeping it off. Consistent behaviors often lead to positive outcomes. To succeed and master anything, you must be consistent with the actions you take daily.

In order to be consistent with your actions, you need to develop a plan that fits you and works for your current situation. Weight-loss strategies are not universal. If you are bouncing around following different diet or workout plans, you could end up causing damage in the long run. Once you develop a plan that fits your needs, take action on that plan daily and don't change it for another.

Success will not come overnight. You must take it one day at a time, one workout at a time, and one meal at a time. Chinese philosopher Lao Tsu said: "The journey of a thousand miles begins with one step." Living an active and healthy lifestyle is a journey.

My coaching clients who got the best results were the ones who consistently followed their plans. My clients who were unsuccessful or did not get the results they hoped for usually failed because of a lack of consistency. They would get off to a great start and then start missing workouts, falling back to unhealthy eating habits, or letting distractions get in the way. After a while, they fall off the plan altogether or eventually just quit.

My personal weight-loss journey was no exception. Consistency played a key role in my journey. I kept the momentum rolling by taking it one day at a time and following through on my plan. Even on the days when I was tired or lacked motivation, I kept taking daily action and followed through on my plan. If I slipped up one day, I would put it behind me and focus on the next day. Consistency is not about being perfect; it's about keeping the momentum rolling and taking the actions to accomplish your goals.

<u>Action Steps</u>

✓ What are some of your daily habits? Take a moment to write down your habits.

✓ Circle the habits that are helpful to you. Place an X next to the habits that may be holding you back.

✓ For any habits you marked with an X, think of some ways you can potentially eliminate or replace these habits.

Positive Self-Talk

When you think about your weight-loss goals, what do you hear your inner voice say? Are your inner thoughts positive or motivating? Are they negative or self-defeating? Your self-talk can be the difference between success and failure.

Everyone has internal dialogue or an inner voice that constantly feeds the thoughts in their head. Depending on what you are going through, this internal dialogue or self-talk may be positive or negative. Most of our self-talk is unconscious; we are not even aware of it, but it will affect and influence what we do in every area of our lives.

Understanding self-talk is so important for your health and fitness. The dialogue or self-talk that takes place will impact your weight-loss goals, either helping you succeed or keeping you paralyzed in fear.

Positive self-talk helps fill your mind and thoughts with positive words or images. It replaces negative thoughts that creep into your mind when faced with adversity or difficult situations.

Positive self-talk uplifts you, helps increase your confidence, enables you to attract what your heart desires, allows you to live a healthier lifestyle, and helps reduce stress.

When negative situations arise, positive self-talk helps bring the positive out of a negative situation to help you feel better, do more, or keep moving toward your goal. The practice of positive self-talk allows you to see the silver lining, truth, hope, and joy in any situation.

One powerful way to improve self-talk is with affirmations. Affirmations are positive statements you write out and/or repeat to yourself to build up self-confidence and belief. Affirmations are personal and should inspire and motivate you to be better and take action.

Affirmations are powerful because they allow you to focus on your goals and desires. In addition, affirmations will position your thoughts to be positive and eliminate self-doubt and self-sabotage. When you write them out or repeat them often, you can reframe your mindset and make positive changes. This is an effective way to reprogram your thoughts and eliminate negative thinking or feelings. Affirmations are written in the present tense, have a positive tone, and are personal.

Present tense - Affirmations are written as if you had already achieved the desired outcome.

Positive - Affirmations are positive. They should inspire and motivate you.

Personal - Affirmations are specific to you. They are not designed for or provided by anyone else.

Affirmations starting with "I am" can be powerful. Below are examples of affirmations I used to reframe my thinking during my weight-loss journey:

- I am happy and thankful!
- I am excellent at what I do!
- I am grateful!
- I am focused!
- I can do this!
- I enjoy exercise!
- I enjoy prepping my meals!
- I am successful!
- I am capable!
- I am lean and fit!

- I am strong!
- I am at peace!
- I am the man!

As you can see, affirmations are powerful and can help you reframe your thoughts. Negative thoughts and feelings will arise, but affirmations will help you conquer those negative thoughts and help you focus on what's important.

Years ago, I learned a person could reprogram their internal dialogue from negative to positive through repetition and practice. The following are four highly effective ways to improve your self-talk.

Action Step - 4 ways to improve your self-talk

✓ The first step is awareness. Pay attention to your thoughts and what you say to yourself. Make note of any negative thoughts or dialogue you have regarding weight loss or fitness. Try to understand what drives those thoughts and feelings.

✓ Replace negative thoughts with positive thoughts. For example, rather than dreading the thought of exercising in the morning, think of the positive benefits and how great you will feel for conquering one of your goals for the day. Instead of beating yourself up over having an unhealthy meal, think about your next healthy meal and tell yourself that one unhealthy meal will not stop you from reaching your goal.

✓ Focus on your goal or what you want as opposed to what you want to avoid or don't want. This approach helps you reframe your thoughts and gets you to focus on the positives rather than the negatives.

✓ Use Affirmations. Affirmations are powerful and go hand in hand with positive self-talk. Affirmations are positive statements that can help you overcome negative thinking.

Eliminating Distractions

Whether you're just getting started with your plan or already executing your goals and living an active and healthy lifestyle, distractions can easily impede or stop your progress. There are so many things that can pop up and pull your attention away from your goals. If you let your guard down, you can get sucked into these time-consuming activities. Time is precious. The way you spend your time has a direct correlation with progress toward goals.

Distractions can come from all areas of your life: home, work, school, etc. The distractions will vary from person to person based on lifestyle and goals. Below are some common distractions to look out for when trying to lose weight and live a healthy lifestyle:

Fad Diets

Many people get sucked into fad diets or the latest "lose weight quick" schemes. These do not provide real or sustainable results. A lot of fad diets make claims that are not supported by research or have not been scientifically proven to be effective. Don't get sucked into the hype. Stick to the basics and focus on healthy lifestyle habits.

Family/Friends/Co-Workers

The people in your life can be a distraction. It's important to consider who you spend your time with and who has influence over your life. It helps tremendously to share your goals and gain as much support as possible, but it's also wise to distance yourself from those who do not support your goals. Be cognizant of your relationships and how they relate to your goal.

Television

According to a recent Nielsen report, the average person spends three to four hours per day watching TV.[4] There are so many good series that are just waiting to be binge-watched. This is another distraction to look out for!

Social Media

There are so many social media platforms and outlets out there. It's easy to get sucked in and waste precious time that could have gone toward your health and fitness goals.

Cell Phone/Internet/Surfing the web

What would we do without our precious cell phones? I think cellphones are one of the greatest inventions ever, but they can also be a distraction if you do not effectively manage your usage throughout the day. Be cautious of the time you are spending talking, using apps, surfing the web, etc. Also, be especially cautious when working out or taking part in physical activity. I often see people in the gym spending more time on the phone than they do working out.

Competing Goals

Competing goals can lead to distractions that impede or halt progress on your goals. For example, let's say you have two goals: the first goal is to gain some muscle mass, and the second goal is to complete a full marathon. It would be counterintuitive to achieve both goals in the same timeframe. The training methods, nutrition needs, and time commitment are at different ends of the spectrum, and the activities to accomplish each goal would pull you in different directions. Which activity takes priority? Choose the one that is most important to you and accomplish that one first before moving on to the second goal.

Luckily, there are ways you can manage and minimize distractions to help you stay focused on your goals:

5 Tips to help reduce or eliminate distractions

1) Prioritize your goals and keep them in front of you

This is key! The things that are most important to you will get the most attention, so your health and fitness goals need to be a top priority. When you are committed to and taking action toward your goals, you will be less likely to get distracted.

2) Plan Ahead

One of my favorite quotes from Benjamin Franklin regarding planning is, "When you fail to plan, you plan to fail."

Not having a plan is a recipe for failure and opens the door for distractions. You can eliminate many distractions by simply making and executing your plan. You should know in advance how you are going to spend your time. This was one of the healthy lifestyle habits that helped me most during my journey.

3) Clear your mind

Your internal and external environment plays a major role. Keep your goals in front of you daily and clear your mind of negative thoughts. If you find yourself preoccupied with thoughts or feelings that prevent you from working on your goals, clear your mind and remember why you started. This would be a wonderful opportunity to review your "why" to get your thoughts and feelings back on track.

4) Control the things you can control

You will not always have control over the things that are external to you. However, you always have control over your actions and how you react to certain situations. For example, there may be polarizing information in your social media feed that may upset you. Instead of reacting negatively, you can choose to ignore the content or take a step back, take a deep breath, and simply move on with your day.

5) Set clear boundaries

This is especially important for your family, friends, co-workers, or anyone you may interact with regularly. You must set clear boundaries in order to manage interactions and get the support you need from those who are close to you, without letting them distract or discourage you. Clear boundaries help define what you are comfortable with regarding your weight-loss plan and how others can support you. For example, a clear boundary I set with my family during my weight-loss journey was to limit eating out to no more than twice a month.

These tips will help you stay on track with your goals. Author James Clear said it best, "Focus is the art of knowing what to ignore."[5] Eliminate those distractions and stay focused!

Reflection

What distractions are you currently dealing with? What can you do today to eliminate those distractions?

5 Ds

Early in my weight-loss journey, I was seeking to understand what it takes to be successful. I recognized there was more to it than exercise and following a healthy diet. The Ds of success is a framework I stumbled across many years ago in an article by Tim O'Brien. His article describes the 7 Ds to success and how they will increase your chances of succeeding in life or your current project.[6] This framework resonated with me and how I think about success. The Ds are characteristics and traits that are put into practice by the most successful men and women. This framework intrigued me and I adopted five of the seven Ds into my life and how I approach success.

The Five Ds are Desire, Dedication, Discipline, Determination, and Drive.

Desire

Your desire comes from within and is the starting point for success. One of the main reasons you are reading this book is because you have a burning desire—perhaps to lose weight or to learn how to live an active and healthy lifestyle. Desire fuels any dream or goal. Your "why" that we discussed earlier in the book speaks directly to your desires. Successful people have a strong desire to succeed and know what they want to accomplish—and why.

I had a burning desire to lose weight and to live an active, healthy lifestyle. I wanted so badly to succeed. My reasons why were strong, and they motivated me enough to commit to the process. I kept the desire burning, keeping my goals in front of me and visualizing what success looks like.

Dedication

When it comes to accomplishing your goals, dedication is one key to success. Without dedication, I wouldn't be the man I am today. I'm dedicated to my wife and children. I'm dedicated to my profession and my business. I'm dedicated to health and fitness—those who know me well know that I am dedicated to living *That Fit Life*! Losing weight and keeping the weight off is difficult, but it is achievable.

My dedication and hard work allowed me to achieve my goals, and now I'm able to promise that your dedication will pay off!

Discipline

Success in any endeavor requires a certain amount of discipline. Success in weight loss requires discipline. Getting your mind right, eating right, and exercising right all require discipline. Discipline is all about doing the things you need to do when you need to do them.

Take a moment to think about all the successful people in your life or those you admire or follow. Do you think these individuals are disciplined when it comes to their talents or gifts? I bet the answer is yes! These individuals are willing to do what it takes to realize their dreams.

I like to think of discipline as "making the right decisions consistently, day after day." Those looking to make healthy lifestyle changes are often faced with many important decisions. When these individuals are consistent in making the right decisions, their odds of achieving their goals will drastically increase.

Determination

Determination is the thing that will keep you on the right track to reach your goal. You know you are determined if you will stop at nothing to reach your goal. You will not let excuses or roadblocks get in your way. You will not let distractions pull you away. You will keep pushing forward, no matter the challenge or obstacle. No matter how many times you get knocked down, you will keep getting back up. That's the power of determination!

Drive

A person with drive is easy to spot! They know what they want, and they know how to get it. If they don't know how to get it, they quickly take action to learn how to get it. A person with drive is self-motivated and a self-starter. They don't need anyone to tell them what to do. A driven person takes full ownership of their actions.

When I think of drive, I always make the comparison to the drive gear in an automobile. In order to move forward, you must take the gear selector and put it in drive. When you throw the other four Ds in the mix, a person with drive will have all the power needed to move forward and succeed.

The five Ds were instrumental in my weight-loss journey. They were also instrumental in my career and allowed me to pursue my passions. I witness these traits in all the successful people I know. If you are looking for some traits to cultivate, I recommend starting with the five Ds.

Action Step

✓ Add the five Ds to your vision board. This will serve as a
  reminder of what it takes to be successful.

Motivation

"Motivation is a fire from within."

- Stephen Covey

Motivation is the force that will keep you moving toward your goals. Your "why" we discussed earlier provides the reason, and motivation provides the fuel. Motivation can be both internal and external. Both types of motivation are beneficial and can help you accomplish your weight-loss goals; however, internal motivation is the most critical for long-term success. The reason is that internal motivation comes from within and is most intimately connected to your wants and desires. Internal motivation is what will keep you going when other people, places, or things are not available to motivate you.

A study in the Journal of the American Medical Association examined different weight-loss plans and found no significant difference between the success rate of one program over another.[7] What they did discover is that a person's motivation to stick with a certain program was much more of a key factor in their success. This is a great example of how important motivation is for weight loss.

During my weight-loss journey, I used several strategies to keep motivated. I had my days where things flowed, and everything seemed to click. I also had days where my motivation was low, and I did not feel inspired to conquer my goals. Below are five helpful strategies I used to boost my motivation.

1) Read goals daily

I had my goals on my vision board, and I also posted them on the refrigerator so I could see them daily. I even wrote my goals on index cards and carried them with me.

2) Read motivational and inspirational quotes daily

I developed the habit of reading motivational and inspirational quotes daily. There is nothing like a good motivational quote or message when things get tough, or when you are low on motivation. I look up quotes online and have motivational posters and calendars posted in my home and workspace.

3) Read health and fitness articles

I read at least one health or fitness article every day. This strategy allows me to build my skills and continue learning about health and fitness. I find I am at my highest motivation levels when I am learning and applying new things.

4) Keep a journal or diary

I kept a journal to track my daily meals, exercise, and other key info. When working with clients, I always recommend they keep a journal to help keep track of progress and to use it as a reflective/motivational tool to show how far they've come. A good example to support this strategy can be found in a study published in the *American Journal for Preventive Medicine*. They found that people who consistently journaled their food intake lost more weight than those that did not.[8]

5) Gain support from family and friends

Sharing your goals with family, friends, and co-workers can help boost both external and internal motivation. You get the external boost by gaining their support and encouragement, and you get the internal boost by holding yourself accountable and making a commitment to those close to you. During my journey, I made sure that everyone closest to me understood my goals and what I was working toward. This helped me tremendously because I received a great deal of support and motivation.

You will encounter challenging days in your journey. The key is knowing how to reignite your own fire and get the momentum rolling again. You have everything within you to succeed.

<u>Dreams</u>

I know what you are thinking: "What do dreams have to do with weight loss and living a healthy lifestyle?"

For some, losing weight is something so far out of reach, it feels like a dream. I was one of those people who dreamed of being lean and fit. When I was at my heaviest, I used to think, "Someday, I'll get the motivation to get off the couch and start losing weight." I'm so glad I kept the dream alive and turned it into a goal.

You must believe in your dream and not let fear hold you back. If you forgot how to dream or need a crash course in using your imagination, hang out with some children. They have dreaming and imagination nailed down to a science. I firmly believe dreaming is healthy for adults, especially when trying to achieve big goals in life. What you need to do is take that dream and bring it into reality by making it a goal, and then put together a plan. Once you have a plan in place, start taking massive action on that plan until you reach your goal.

If not for my daughters, Teairra and Lakeya, I would have not written this book. They are both at the age where their imaginations run wild, and anything is possible. I constantly feed into this magical mind power and allow myself to imagine and dream with them. My vision board is filled with all my major goals and dreams. I have my vision board visible in my loft where anyone can view it. I'm not ashamed to put my wild ideas out there and to dream big. What matters is my belief and how I pursue those dreams.

Reflection

What motivates you when it comes to losing weight and living an active and healthy lifestyle?

What are your major goals and dreams?

Self-Awareness

Having self-awareness means having a clear understanding of who you are and how you relate to other people. Self-awareness is important in all aspects of life, including personal, family, and professional. It's especially important for your health and fitness goals.

As I grow better (not older) and wiser, I have become a firm believer that self-awareness is a critical component of achieving success. Having strong self-awareness will allow you to understand your strengths and weaknesses.

Self-awareness starts with understanding your own strengths and weaknesses. Leveraging your strengths and improving on your weaknesses will yield great benefits in your weight-loss journey. For example, you may have strengths in cooking and meal prep but be inexperienced with weight training. You may have minimal knowledge in reading nutrition labels but are skilled in taking body measurements. The key is knowing where you stand and what areas to leverage.

Along with understanding your strengths and weaknesses, it's important to practice self-reflection. Self-reflection allows you to learn from your experiences. In addition, self-reflection allows you to gain a better understanding of yourself, your life, and the people in your life.

Another component I would like to mention regarding the importance of self-awareness is feedback. Seeking and being open to honest feedback—both positive and constructive—is vital when it comes to self-awareness. Feedback has played a significant role in my growth and development as a husband, father, and professional.

Mastery of Self

Mastery of Self is the process of continuous personal growth and development. It is the ability to strive for your highest potential or major goals in life.

In the early days of struggling with my weight, I had very little knowledge of nutrition and fitness. In addition, I did not understand my body or the behaviors that caused weight gain.

Since then, I have learned that if you want to lose weight and live an active and healthy lifestyle, you must work on changing your behaviors. In order to change your behaviors, you must educate yourself, set SMART goals, and take the right action. You must start where you are and intentionally build from there. In essence, you must work toward building the best version of you.

I have "Mastery of Self" written on my vision board, and it has been there since day one. It serves as a reminder to continue improving and growing so that I can reach my full potential and continue accomplishing my major goals in life.

Reflection

Do you know your strengths and weaknesses as they relate to your weight-loss goals? Please take a moment to reflect on your strengths and weaknesses and write them down.

Believe in Yourself

If you can read these words, you have everything you need to succeed. You have breath in your body, and you are alive. You are enough, and you must believe in yourself.

Believing in yourself is a key ingredient when embarking on any journey, especially the weight-loss journey. Belief will guide your dreams, thoughts, and actions. Belief will keep you going when things get tough and when adversity comes your way. Belief will be the fuel that gets you out of bed in the morning, helps you make that healthy meal, and gets you into the gym to work out. You must believe in your current abilities, and you must believe that you can develop and learn new abilities.

Early in my journey, I had trouble believing in myself and my abilities. I was always making excuses for why I would not take action or could not reach my goals. I often felt like I did not have enough information or resources to commit to my goals. I was missing something. That something was belief in myself.

Several studies have shown that when dieters believe they can lose weight, they have a higher chance of reaching their goal.

There is a special term for the way you believe in your ability to reach your goal: self-efficacy. The American Council on Exercise defines self-efficacy as "One's perception of his or her ability to change or to perform specific behaviors."[9] There is a strong link between self-efficacy and success in weight loss.

In other words, if you believe you can be healthier, you will be.

Do you believe in yourself? Here are three ways to build your belief in yourself and to get you set up for success:

1) Examine your thoughts - Are your thoughts positive or negative? Do you have limiting beliefs that hold you back? Are you holding on to thoughts or beliefs that may not be true? It's important to examine your thoughts and to clear any negative or limiting beliefs.

2) Focus on quick wins - Take small steps and accomplish a few of your short-term goals to help build confidence in your abilities. It can be as simple as completing your first workout or prepping your next healthy meal.

3) Learn and apply a new skill that will aid you on your journey - It's amazing how the learning process can spark creativity and build confidence. Some examples that will aid in your weight-loss journey could be attending a healthy-cooking class, trying a new group fitness class at the gym, or learning how to meditate.

Chapter 1 Summary

◇ Before starting this fit-life journey, it's important to understand your "why."

◇ If you are serious about reaching your goal, you must make a commitment.

◇ Goal setting is an extremely important step when trying to achieve any type of success in life. Goals provide direction and help guide your actions.

◇ Structuring your goals using the SMART approach will allow you to achieve great success.

◇ The main purpose of the vision board is to serve as a symbolic source for inspiration and motivation.

◇ Habits can make you or break you when it comes to living a healthy lifestyle.

◇ Positive self-talk uplifts you, helps increase your confidence, enables you to attract what your heart desires, allows you to adopt a healthier lifestyle, and helps reduce stress.

◇ Affirmations are powerful because they allow you to focus on your goals and desires. In addition, affirmations will position your thoughts to be positive and eliminate self-doubt and self-sabotage.

◇ Motivation can be both internal and external. Both types of motivation are beneficial and can help you accomplish your weight-loss goals.

Chapter 1 Summary

◇ Consistency is not about being perfect; it's about keeping the momentum rolling and taking action to accomplish your goals.

◇ Self-awareness starts with understanding your own strengths and weaknesses. Leveraging your strengths and improving on your weaknesses will yield great benefits in your weight-loss journey.

◇ You must believe in your dream and not let fear hold you back.

◇ Belief will guide your dreams, thoughts, and actions.

Chapter 2
Nutrition Pillar

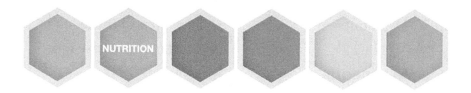

"The doctor of the future will no longer treat the human frame with drugs, but will rather cure and prevent disease with nutrition."

- Thomas Edison

Chapter 2 Introduction

The next Pillar we are going to explore is the Nutrition Pillar. Nutrition is essential for life and is extremely important for weight loss. Weight loss will be an uphill battle if you do not understand the basics. The Nutrition Pillar focuses on how to design a nutrition plan that works best for you.

In this chapter, we are going to dive into the following topics:

• The Law of Calorie Balance	• Meal Quantity
• Macronutrients	• Improve Food Quality
• Micronutrients	• Limit these foods
• MyPlate	• Eat more of these foods!
• Glycemic Index	• Eat Less/Exercise more
• Meal Prep	• Types of Diets
• 80/20 Rule & Free Days	• Diets are not a one size fits all

The best diet is one you can stick with consistently and make a part of your lifestyle. The Nutrition Pillar will highlight the keys needed to make the right changes for long-term success.

I've learned, in my 20-year journey, that changes don't happen overnight. The best approach is to make small changes over time. Just as we discussed in the Mental chapter, it's better to focus on consistency instead of perfection.

The Law of Calorie Balance

You can't outrun a bad diet! Good nutrition starts with a solid understanding of calories, protein, fats, carbohydrates, and the impacts of these macronutrients on your diet. When it comes to nutrition goals, it is not "one size fits all." Nutrition must be customized based on your specific goals and body type.

The first topic we are going to cover in the Nutrition Pillar is the law of calorie balance, which helps set the foundation when discussing nutrition and goal setting.

Calories

By definition, a calorie is "the amount of energy needed to increase one kilogram of water by one degree Celsius."[1] In other words, a calorie is a measure of energy. This energy is released from food during the digestion process. The macronutrients protein, carbohydrates, and fat contain calories. Fat provides nine calories per gram. Carbohydrates and protein each contain four calories per gram.

Calorie Balance

Calorie balance is the relationship between calories consumed and calories burned by your body through exercise and other activities. This is a very important relationship to understand. Your ability to meet your weight and nutrition goals will heavily depend on how you manage this relationship. Think of calorie balance as an equation, with calories consumed on one side and calories burned on the other side.

- To maintain your weight, the calories you consume must equal the calories you burn: Calories Consumed (calories in) = Calories Burned (calories out)
- To lose weight, you must burn more calories than you consume: Calories Consumed < Calories Burned
- To gain weight, you must consume more calories than you burn: Calories Consumed > Calories Burned

Respect the law of
Calorie Balance!

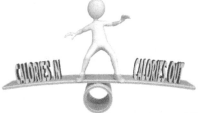

Want to Lose Weight?	Want To Maintain Weight?	Want to Gain Weight?
Calories in < Calories Out	Calories in = Calories Out	Calories in > Calories Out
Goal is to create a Calorie Deficit	Goal is to balance Calories	Goal is to create a Calorie Surplus

During my transformation, I paid close attention to the calorie balance equation. Since my goal was weight loss, it was important that I maintain a steady calorie deficit each week. There are approximately 3,500 calories in one pound of stored fat. In order to lose one pound, you need to burn 3,500 calories through diet, exercise, or a combination of both. For safe weight loss, you should aim to lose only one to two pounds per week, which means you should have a deficit of 3,500-7,000 calories per week. If you try to lose more than two pounds per week, you are at risk of burning muscle mass and decreasing your metabolism.[2]

Calorie Requirements

Now let's discuss calorie requirements. In order to manage the calorie balance equation, you need to know how many calories your body requires. Calorie requirements will vary from person to person due to gender, age, height, weight, body composition, and other factors. For example, my daily calorie requirements to maintain my current weight are approximately 2,900 calories. This same 2,900 calories would be a surplus for my wife because her maintenance requirement is 2,400 calories.

Calorie requirements are calculated by taking your Basal Metabolic Rate (BMR) and multiplying it by a specific activity factor. The result is your Total Daily Energy Expenditure (TDEE). Your BMR is the number of calories you burn while your body is at rest. This is the number of calories needed for basic bodily function. Your TDEE is an estimation of how many calories you burn per day with activity factored in. "Activity" is comprised of two components: exercise and non-exercise activity.

There are several calorie calculators and formulas on the web that provide a very good estimate of calorie requirements. Most of the good calculators base the requirements on your basal metabolic rate and an activity factor. A good website to reference is www.bmi-calculator.net.[3]

For those that want to see the math behind the calculators (I love math), here are two good equations I used to calculate BMR. The first equation is the Harris-Benedict equation. The equation is different for men and women.[4]

The Harris-Benedict equation for men:

- BMR = 66 + (13.7 x weight in kilograms) + (5 x height in centimeters) - (6.8 x age in years)

The Harris-Benedict equation for women:

- BMR = 655 + (9.6 x weight in kilograms) + (1.8 x height in centimeters) - (4.7 x age in years)

As you can see, the Harris-Benedict equation for determining BMR factors in weight, height, and age. Most calculators on the web use this formula for their calculations. If you ever wondered how the calculators determined your BMR, now you can verify the accuracy.

The second equation is the Katch-McArdle equation. The equation is the same for both men and women. This equation factors in lean mass, which can be determined if you know your body-fat percentage.[5]

Katch-McArdle equation: BMR = 370 + (21.6 x lean mass in kilograms).

Both equations do a great job estimating BMR. The Katch-McArdle is slightly more accurate because it factors in lean mass.

Once you determine your BMR, you can calculate your TDEE by applying an activity multiplier.

Activity Multiplier:

- Sedentary - BMR x 1.2 (little or no exercise)
- Lightly active - BMR x 1.375 (light exercise 1-3 days/week)

- Moderately active - BMR x 1.55 (moderate exercise 3-5 days/week)
- Very active - BMR x 1.725 (hard exercise 6-7 days/week)
- Extremely active - BMR x 1.9 (hard daily exercise or training twice per day)

Here is an example of my TDEE using the Katch-McArdle equation to determine my BMR and using the moderately active multiplier.

BMR = 370 + (21.6 x 72 kg) = 1925.2

Calorie requirements = 1925.2 x 1.55 (since I'm moderately active) = 2984

Understanding calorie balance is key for you to establish the right SMART goal for weight loss. Once you know your TDEE, you can create a safe calorie deficit that will allow you to lose between one to two pounds per week. Now that you have a good understanding of calorie balance, let's cover macronutrients.

Action Steps - Determine your BMR and TDEE

✓ Using one of the BMR equations, calculate your BMR.

✓ Once you determine your BMR, calculate your TDEE using one of the activity multipliers.

Macronutrients

The macronutrients protein, carbohydrates, and fat play a vital role in nutrition. There are good types of all of them and types to avoid. The key is knowing the difference and choosing the right food combinations.

Protein

Protein is an important macronutrient. In my opinion, it is the most important when it comes to exercise and nutrition. Proteins contain four calories per gram and are the building blocks for cells in the body. They play a critical role in many bodily functions, including but not limited to:

- Building, repairing, and strengthening of cells
- Carrying oxygen in the blood
- Carrying vitamins, nutrients, and iron in the blood
- Producing hormones and enzymes
- Strengthening immunity
- Maintaining balanced blood-sugar levels

Proteins are made from amino acids, and your body can produce most of the amino acids found in protein. "Non-essential" amino acids can be produced or synthesized in the body, while "essential" amino acids come only from food or supplements and cannot be generated in the body.

The most common protein sources are meats, poultry, fish, seafood, and eggs, which are all "complete" proteins. Complete proteins contain all essential amino acids. Nuts, vegetables, grains, and fruit contain some protein; however, most do not contain all essential amino acids and are therefore "incomplete" proteins.

When choosing proteins, it is best to choose lean proteins. Lean proteins contain fewer calories overall and less total fat. Eat a variety of lean proteins every week and use various healthy cooking methods like grilling, broiling, roasting, or baking. Here is a listing of my "go-to" lean proteins I eat regularly.

- Chicken breast
- Turkey breast
- Ground turkey
- Fish (salmon, perch, tuna, cod)
- Shrimp
- Lean ground beef
- Lean beef
- Lean pork
- Egg whites
- Whole eggs
- Whey protein

Carbohydrates

I like to think of carbohydrates as the primary fuel for the body, as they are the body's preferred energy source. Like protein, carbohydrates contain four calories per gram. Carbohydrates fall into two major categories: complex carbohydrates and simple carbohydrates. Complex carbohydrates consist of sugar molecules that are strung together in long complex chains. Simple carbohydrates consist of only one or two sugar molecules. Complex carbohydrates are often rich in fiber, while simple carbohydrates contain little fiber.

Examples of complex carbohydrates:

- Brown rice
- Green vegetables
- Fruit
- Whole grains
- Oatmeal
- Quinoa
- Sweet potatoes
- Corn
- Beans
- Peas
- Whole-grain bread

Examples of simple carbohydrates:

- Sugar
- Corn syrup
- High fructose corn syrup
- Jelly
- Candy
- Soda/soft drinks
- Fruit drinks
- White rice
- White bread
- Cookies
- Donuts

When choosing carbohydrates, it is best to choose complex carbohydrates. Complex carbohydrates provide vitamins, minerals, and fiber, which are essential for overall health.

Simple carbohydrates do not contain vitamins, minerals, or fiber, and many of them have little to no nutritional value.

Choose whole or unprocessed foods from plant sources whenever possible. This comes down to making simple substitutions with your meals—for example, choose whole-grain bread instead of white bread, or quinoa instead of white rice. The goal is to make healthier choices.

Fats

Fat is the most energy-dense of the macronutrients. Fat contains nine calories per gram, which is 2.25 times more calories than protein and carbohydrates. Like protein, fat plays a critical role in many bodily functions, including but not limited to the following:

- Provide energy (stored energy)
- Insulation
- Vitamin absorption
- Regulate production of hormones
- Produce healthy cells

There are five different types of fat. Three of the types (monounsaturated fatty acids, polyunsaturated fatty acids, and omega-3 fatty acids) are beneficial, while two types (saturated fat and trans-fat) are harmful when consumed in high amounts.

Examples of food containing healthy fats:

- Fish
- Avocados
- Extra virgin olive oil
- Coconut oil

- Sesame oil
- Flaxseed oil
- Seeds
- Nuts

Macronutrients are the key building blocks of your diet. You are in full control of what types you consume and the amount. One revelation I had during my weight-loss journey was that I was in full control of what I put into my body. I realized it all came down to the choices I made.

__Reflection__

What are some of your favorite healthy proteins, carbs, and fats? How often do you include them in your meals?

Micronutrients

In the previous topic, we learned about macronutrients and the vital role they play in nutrition. Micronutrients—vitamins and minerals—also play a vital role, as they are one of the major groups of nutrients that your body needs to function properly.

We need vitamins and minerals in our diet, and when micronutrients are consumed in the right amounts, they lead to optimal health outcomes. This is especially important for weight loss. When there is a deficiency, our health can be negatively impacted. The World Health Organization (WHO) states micronutrients' "impact on a body's health are critical, and deficiency in any of them can cause severe and even life-threatening conditions."[6] Below is a high-level breakdown of the different types of vitamins and minerals.

Vitamins

Vitamins are organic micronutrients that are essential for normal bodily function. Most vitamins are consumed through the foods we eat. There are two main types of vitamins: water-soluble and fat-soluble.

Water-soluble vitamins are vitamins that dissolve in water. These vitamins cannot be stored in the body and are easily excreted in our urine. This factor decreases the risk of toxicity due to overconsumption. All the B Vitamins (B1, B2, B3, B5, B6, B7, B9, and B12) and vitamin C are water-soluble.

Fat-Soluble Vitamins are found in fat-containing foods. Unlike water-soluble vitamins, fat-soluble vitamins can be stored in the body—in the liver and other fatty tissues. It's important to not over-consume these types of vitamins, due toxicity concerns. In other words, there is a specific limit that is safe for the body. Vitamins A, D, E, and K are the fat-soluble vitamins.

Minerals

Minerals are inorganic micronutrients that are essential for normal body health and function. Minerals are made in the body and found in the food we eat. There are two types of minerals: Macro Minerals and Micro Minerals.

Macro Minerals are minerals that are needed in large amounts. Macro Minerals include calcium, phosphorus, magnesium, sulfur, sodium, chloride, and potassium.

Micro Minerals are called trace minerals. Trace minerals are needed in small amounts. Micro Minerals include copper, fluoride, iron, iodine, manganese, selenium, and zinc.

All foods contain micronutrients, but when choosing healthy food options, the goal is to include foods that are nutrient-dense—in other words, foods that are rich in micronutrients. Doing so helped me establish healthier eating habits during my weight-loss journey. Learning more about micronutrients—and food in general—will help you improve your overall health.

Action Step - Dive Deeper!

✓ For more information on vitamins and minerals, please check out the fact sheets provided by the National Institute of Health (NIH): https://ods.od.nih.gov/factsheets/list-all/

✓ Identify any key vitamins or minerals missing from your diet.

MyPlate

Did you know they replaced the food pyramid with a plate? This change occurred in 2011. The website choosemyplate.gov provides basic nutritional guidelines for Americans. MyPlate provides useful tips and guidelines on healthy eating. It's also a resource that helps you find your healthy eating style and how to build it throughout your lifetime.

The goal of MyPlate is to simplify the USDA nutrition message into an easy-to-understand infographic. The graphic is a dinner plate divided into four sections: fruits, vegetables, protein, grains, and a glass of milk to represent dairy. See graphic below[7]

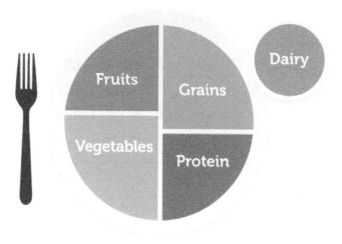

(Image Source:MyPlate.gov)

According to U.S. Department of Agriculture Food and Nutrition Service, MyPlate encourages people to:
- Focus on variety, amount, and nutrition
- Choose foods and beverages with less saturated fat, sodium, and added sugars

- Start with small changes to build healthier eating habits
- Support healthy eating for everyone[8]

MyPlate is a solid base of nutritional information that is backed by research and credible industry sources, and it is a good place to go when you are just getting started with making healthy lifestyle changes. This was a "go to" during my weight-loss journey, and I recommend MyPlate to everyone I work with. MyPlate can help develop individualized eating plans for all walks of life. I keep a picture of MyPlate on my wall as a reminder to make healthy food choices when planning my meals.

Action Step

✓ Go to MyPlate website and take the quiz and get a personalized MyPlate plan. For more information on MyPlate, please check out the following site:

https://www.myplate.gov

Glycemic Index

I learned about the glycemic index many years ago. My father had Type II Diabetes and had several books and pamphlets around the house on diabetes. One topic from those books that stuck out to me at the time was the glycemic index. I'll try not to get too technical with the glycemic index, but I do want to hit some key points and discuss how it can aid in weight loss.

The glycemic index (GI) measures the increase in blood glucose levels after consuming a particular food. This usually applies to carbohydrate-type foods. The index provides a breakdown of high, medium, and low GI food based on how they increase blood glucose levels. Foods with a GI number below 56 are considered low, 56-69 are medium, and 70 or above are high.[9] Comparing these values when choosing carbohydrate foods can help guide healthier food choices. This fits well with eating a healthy diet and with meal preparation.

A diet containing low GI carbohydrates is beneficial for weight loss and weight maintenance. During my weight-loss journey, I used the glycemic index to help make healthy food choices when selecting carbs. By using the index, I could determine which carbs to avoid and which carbs to incorporate into my diet. For example, based on the info in the glycemic index, I swapped out white rice with brown rice because brown rice has a lower GI value and is much healthier compared to white rice.

Studying the GI index, I learned that most complex carbs I enjoy eating have a lower GI value than the value of simple carbs (ex. brown rice GI value: 54 vs white rice GI value: 100, whole-grain bread GI value: 51 vs white bread GI value:100).

When it comes to weight loss, incorporating complex carbs into the diet is the way to go. In addition, low GI foods fall within the MyPlate nutrition guidelines discussed in the previous section.

I hope you find this information to be useful and can now see how this can benefit you when making healthy food choices. This information will help guide your carbohydrate selections for meal preparation.

__Action Steps__

✓ Make a list of your favorite carbohydrate foods.

✓ Look up the GI value of each food and determine if the food is a high, medium, or low GI food. Use this helpful database to find the GI value of each carbohydrate food:

Link - http://www.glycemicindex.com/foodSearch.php

Meal Preparation

"If you keep good food in your fridge, you will eat good food."

- Errick McAdams

Maintaining a healthy diet can be challenging when you are strapped for time or do not have healthy food options available in your home. Meal preparation (or "meal prep") is an effective way to prepare healthy meals ahead of time and control food intake.

Meal preparation is a very important skill to develop for successful weight loss, weight maintenance, or when trying to gain lean muscle mass. Meal prep is all about planning ahead. It's a smart strategy, as it frees up time and energy you would otherwise expend trying to figure out what to eat. Once the food is prepped and packaged, you will have healthy meals that are ready and available whenever you need them.

Meal preparation involves planning your meals ahead of time, going grocery shopping, preparing the food to be cooked, cooking the food, and then storing the food. There's flexibility with meal prep too—you can prepare meals for one day or do multi-day meal prep. You can also prepare full meals at once or prepare proteins and sides separately. The choice is yours.

Below are some key benefits of meal prep, followed by my simple seven-step process.

Plan meals - Meal prep provides you with the opportunity to plan healthy meals, all while giving you the freedom to select the types of protein, carbs, and healthy fats you like or would like to try. Planning meals and trying new recipes are two of my favorite aspects of meal planning.

Control portions and macros - With meal prep, you can better control portion sizes and your macronutrient ratios. There are various food containers and food measuring tools available that can help with portion control and macronutrients.

Save Time - Meal prep streamlines the process and frees up time in your week. When your food is already prepared, cooked, and stored in a meal container, you can just grab and go without thinking about what you need to eat.

Save Money - Having food prepared at home will help you save money by reducing the need to eat out at restaurants. I save about $55 a week by just prepping my own meals for lunch.

Action Steps - 7 step process for meal prep

✓ Gather or review healthy recipes

✓ Create a healthy food shopping list

✓ Go to the grocery and purchase items on the list

✓ Clean and prepare cooking area

✓ Prepare Food

✓ Cook Food

✓ Store food in meal containers

✓ Enjoy!

Meal Quantity

How many meals should I eat per day? This is a question I get asked often. The answer really depends on your goals and current eating habits. Most people land between three and six meals per day. Some people stick with the traditional breakfast, lunch, and dinner (three meals), while others fall below or outside this range. There is no magic number, but it takes a little experimentation to see what works best for you. Again, there is not a one-size-fits-all model; the right number for you is the number of meals you consistently stick with and can sustain over the long term to meet your goals. The focus should be on lifestyle changes versus short-term quick fixes.

Meal frequency studies have shown that there is no significant difference between eating three larger meals per day and eating six small-portion meals in terms of metabolism and general health. In terms of weight loss, the difference really comes down to the overall number of calories consumed.[10]

My sweet spot is six small meals per day. I like to structure my meals and spread them out (one every two to three hours) to prevent hunger and stabilize my blood sugar. I find this approach to be highly effective in reducing food cravings and supporting my active and healthy lifestyle. I structure each meal to include a protein, complex carb, and a healthy fat.

With six meals as my target, my meals are smaller; I adjust my portions and macros based on my calorie goals. This approach was effective during my weight-loss journey, and I continue to use this approach. I start my day with breakfast around 6 a.m. I never skip breakfast. A healthy breakfast kick-starts your metabolism and gets your nutrition on the right track.

Reflection

Based on your own experience, do you prefer smaller, more frequent meals throughout the day, or do you prefer larger, less frequent meals?

Are you willing to experiment to see which approach works best to aid your weight loss or sustain your weight loss?

Do you eat breakfast daily? If not, what time is your first meal of the day?

80/20 Rule & Free Days

In my years of trial and error with food and nutrition, I've found that the 80/20 rule works very well for consistent weight loss and for weight maintenance after you reach your goal. Eighty percent of your meals should be healthy, while 20 percent can be less healthy. This approach provides flexibility with your diet and allows you to continue eating foods you enjoy on your free days. In the next section, I provide more details on free days and how you can incorporate them into your diet. In fact, free days are an integral part of a good nutrition plan. They can be very beneficial as they provide you with more freedom over the long term.

Over the years of my weight-loss journey, I kept track of the number of days I ate clean and the number of free days (aka cheat days) that I had in my food diary. Having this information on hand to review and study gave me some significant insights into my weight-loss results. I was surprised to find that I had better results when I was less restrictive compared to the times when I tried to be 100 percent compliant with my diet. In fact, I found that the more restrictive I was, the more likely I was to abandon or stop following the plan.

I found that I achieved the best results when my adherence was in the 80 percent range. In this range, I found it easy to stay on track over a longer period and I did not feel as though I was deprived of my favorite foods. In addition, this approach improved my overall meal planning and made it less stressful. For example, using this approach, I could plan my free days each month. If my family had to do some traveling or take a vacation,

I could plan for these days without stressing about how I was going to eat or stay on track with my diet. This approach was key in my weight-loss journey and worked extremely well with weight maintenance.

Free Days

Free days are "planned" cheat days or days you can use if you need to break "free" from your nutrition plan. These are the days where you can be more flexible with your diet. If you want a burger, go for it. Cookies? Absolutely! You can use your free days however you like. The key, however, is to not overdo it, or binge eat on these days. I used to be that guy who would avoid family gatherings because I did not want to ruin my diet. In those instances where I did attend, I would not eat anything—or only opt for eating something healthy, if it was available. Ever since I started using the free day approach, it has improved many aspects of my life. Now, I don't have to miss out on family or social gatherings.

This approach has many benefits and is sustainable over the long term. It gives you more flexibility with your nutrition rather than forcing you to be perfect with your nutrition. I've tried many diets in the past that were very restrictive. They may have worked for a brief period; however, they were not sustainable over the long term. You will hear me say this often: it's not about perfection; it's all about consistency.

One last thing: with this approach, you do not have to take all your free days. There will be some months where you use only a couple of your free days, and that is perfectly fine.

Reflection

What do you think of this approach?

Is this something you can implement as part of a nutrition plan and healthy lifestyle?

Would four to six free days per month give you the flexibility to plan around holidays, vacations, or other life situations that may pop up?

Improve Food Quality

Improving the quality of foods that you eat must be a top priority for healthy living. You start where you are by replacing unhealthy food with healthy food options. For example, swap out those potato chips for a piece of fresh fruit. Swap the soda for water or green tea. These small improvements in your nutrition will have a positive effect on your health and help you reach your weight-loss goals.

Researchers at the Harvard School of Public Health conducted a study that suggests choosing high-quality foods over lower-quality foods is an important factor in helping people consume fewer calories.[11] Making those incremental swaps in your diet will have a positive impact.

Improving food quality takes time and patience. The key is to choose a variety of food that you like. There are so many healthy food options to explore and customize to fit your preferences. I try not to fall into the trap of prescribing a certain diet or restricting to certain foods—for example, having a plan that suggests you need to eat broccoli every day. I hate broccoli. How long do you think I would adhere to that plan? Not very long. However, there are other healthy vegetable options I do like that are just as healthy as broccoli.

Next, we'll cover the foods you should limit, as well as the foods you should eat more of.

Reflection

Can you think of any food items that you would like to swap out for healthier options? You don't have to swap out all items at once. You can start with one item at a time and work at your own pace.

Limit these foods!

Some foods, when eaten in excessive quantities, can have a negative impact on your diet and can lead to weight gain. We all know what those foods are—the same foods we've been warned about since we were kids, from our teachers, our parents, television, radio, the internet, social media...the list goes on. These foods lack nutritional value and have high amounts of unhealthy fat and sugar, which end up tipping the scale on us when it comes to the law of calorie balance.

I've analyzed the foods that were in my diet when I was overweight, as well as the diets of my clients, friends, and family. What I learned over the years is that most overweight individuals who struggle with nutrition over-consume foods that fall into the following categories:

Highly Processed Food - Processed foods are foods that are packaged, boxed, frozen, canned, dried, baked, or pasteurized. Highly processed foods can contain high amounts of sugar, sodium, oil, additives, and preservatives

Junk Food - Unhealthy food high in calories from sugar and fat that contains very limited nutritional value; examples include candy bars, potato chips, cookies

Fried Food - Foods that are fried in grease or oil; examples - French fries, fried chicken, onion rings, cheese sticks

Fast Food - Food prepared and served quickly from fast-food restaurants

Foods that contain a high amount of high fructose corn syrup - Sweetener made from cornstarch mainly found in sugary drinks and processed foods; example - soda, crackers, cakes, cookies

Food that contains high amounts of trans fat - a type of unsaturated fat found in processed foods or snacks; examples - crackers, cookies, fast foods

These are the foods you want to limit or avoid when trying to lose weight. They should also be limited to prevent chronic illness or even prevent death. When eaten frequently or in excess for a long period, these foods can lead to serious health problems down the road. A study published in the Lancet Journal provided evidence that suggested poor diets are the leading risk factor for deaths in many countries around the world.[12] This is very alarming!

The key to turning this around is to continue educating yourself and to live an active and healthy lifestyle. If you follow recommendations from MyPlate, develop a clean eating approach, and improve food quality over time, you'll be well on your way to losing weight and improving your lifestyle.

Action Step

✓ Make a list of the top five foods you are over consuming. Compare your list to the categories of foods to limit.

Eat more of these foods!

We just covered the foods to limit or avoid for weight loss and healthy living. So, the million-dollar question is, what foods should we eat more of? Below are some of the "go-to" foods for successful weight loss and healthy living.

Fruits & Vegetables

Fruits and vegetables should be at the heart of any healthy diet. There are many types to choose from, and it's important to include a variety to ensure you are getting vitamins, minerals, and antioxidants.

Whole Grains

Whole grains are a necessity in a healthy diet. Natural and minimally processed whole grains are a good source of fuel and, when eaten regularly, can help lower the risk of obesity. Whole grains include barley, corn, rice, wheat, quinoa, and rye, just to name a few. Whole grains also contain antioxidants, vitamins, and minerals.

Lean Protein

Lean proteins are foods rich in protein and low in fat. Eating lean protein is beneficial for a healthy diet and for weight loss. Lean protein is instrumental for building and maintaining muscle. Lean protein includes chicken breast, fish, turkey, lean meats (beef, pork), beans, lentils, egg whites, low-fat cottage cheese, and Greek yogurt. A high protein intake helps boost the metabolism, reduce appetite, and aid in weight loss.

Healthy Fats

As we learned earlier, fats are one of the three essential macronutrients that the body needs to function properly. A healthy diet should include healthy (monounsaturated and polyunsaturated) fats. Some of the best sources of these types of fats are found in avocados, fish, olive oil, nuts, seeds, flaxseed, and other oils made from plants or seeds. Including healthy fats in your diet helps reduce the risk of heart disease and helps lower cholesterol.

Low-fat or fat-free dairy

Remember the slogan "Milk does the body good"? Dairy foods are a good source of protein and contain both vitamins and minerals. When choosing dairy, it is best to choose low-fat or fat-free to avoid additional amounts of saturated fat. As we covered earlier in the book (in the MyPlate section), dairy is one of the key food groups to include in a healthy and balanced diet.

Nuts & Seeds

Nuts and seeds play a key role in a healthy diet. They contain antioxidants, fiber, vitamins, and minerals. In addition, nuts contain the healthy fats that we touched on above. We can add nuts and seeds to salads, smoothies, or eaten by themselves as snacks throughout the day.

Reflection

Which of these foods are you eating plenty of? Which of these foods do you need to eat more of to round out your diet?

Eat less/Exercise more

If I had to sum up everything I learned over the years about weight loss and put it into one sentence or phrase, it would be to Eat Less and Exercise More. That's it! You can put the book down and have a solid game plan for an active and healthy lifestyle.

...It's much easier said than done, isn't it?

But when you think about it, losing weight is really that simple. It's when you factor in this thing called "life" that things get a little complicated. In addition, all the information floating around out there about the "best diets" and "best exercises" can make it even more confusing. Now that you have a basic understanding of the fundamentals and the law of calorie balance, you can save a lot of frustration in the long run by starting off on the right foot.

The most effective way to create a calorie deficit and lose weight is to reduce the number of calories you consume (eat less) and increase the number of calories you burn (exercise more). You can accomplish the "eat less" part by finding a diet that works best for you—one that you can stick with over the long term. As for the "exercise more" part, incorporate both weight training and cardio into your plan. We'll dive more into exercise in the following chapter, but for now, let's get your diet squared away.

<u>Reflection</u>

Think about the last time you were on a diet or following a nutrition plan. What were some of the elements that worked well? What were some of the elements that did not work well for you? Based on what you learned so far, what would you do differently moving forward?

Types of Diets

There are so many diets out there, and just as many experts or gurus making a case for why their certain diet is better than others. All diets have their pros and cons, and they all work to some extent for weight loss, especially when there is a calorie deficit.

In this section, I will provide a short list of some of the popular mainstream diets out there. I tried many of them over the years, and some worked better than others. Take this as further evidence that one diet does not fit all with nutrition, and that the best diet is the diet you can stick to.

The Paleo Diet

The Paleo diet is based on the premise of eating as the Paleolithic humans ate. The basic concept of the Paleo diet is to eat only whole foods and avoid processed foods.

Ketogenic Diet (Keto)

Keto, a very low-carb, high-fat diet, is a very popular diet right now. The basic concept of the keto diet is to get your body in a metabolic state called ketosis. Ketosis involves the body producing ketone bodies out of fat and using fat for energy instead of carbohydrates.

Low-Fat Diet

A low-fat diet is a diet where only 30 percent of the calories come from fat. Low-fat diets usually call for restricting foods high in saturated fat and cholesterol.

Low-Carb Diet

A low-carb diet is a diet where carb intake is reduced to 150 grams or fewer. These diets are usually higher in protein with a moderate amount of fat.

High Protein

A high protein diet is a diet where 30-40 percent of the calories are from protein. The concept behind high protein diets is that they decrease hunger and increase feelings of fullness, resulting in eating less food overall. The diets also help build, protect, and prevent muscle loss.

The Mediterranean Diet

The Mediterranean Diet is a diet based on the cuisines typically found in countries bordering the Mediterranean Sea. The diet includes plant-based foods, whole grains, healthy fats, and seafood.

The South Beach Diet

The South Beach Diet is a low-carb diet created by cardiologist Dr. Arthur Agatston. The diet focuses on lean meats, healthy fats, and low-glycemic carbs.

The Vegetarian Diet

Vegetarian diets eliminate meat, fish, poultry, eggs, and dairy products. A healthy vegetarian diet includes fruits and vegetables, legumes, nuts, and whole grains. Some people may choose to adopt a vegetarian lifestyle for religion, environmental benefits, or to support animal rights. For example, they may avoid products that are made from animals like fur or leather.

The Vegan Diet

Vegan diets are made up of only plant-based foods. They do not include animal foods or animal byproducts.

There are many diets that will support you in your weight-loss journey. Eating healthy does not have to be complicated. It comes down to knowing the basics and incorporating healthy eating habits. There is plenty of flexibility for you to create a plan that includes the healthy foods you enjoy.

Reflection

Review the list and see if you recognize any of the diets. Have you followed any of the diets? Have any of the diets worked well for you in the past? Is there a diet on the list you would like to try?

Diets are not one-size-fits-all

When it comes to your health and fitness goals, nutrition is not a "one size fits all." Your nutrition plan must be customized based on your specific goals and body type. We must stop thinking about short-term diets and start thinking about healthy lifestyle changes. Anyone can follow a strict diet for a little while, but if you can't stick with it long-term or adopt it into your lifestyle, what's the point?

The diet that works best for you is the one that provides you with the best results. In other words, the best diet is one you can stick with over the long term. Plain and simple. Having a clear picture of your goals and understanding how your body responds to the types of food you put in it is essential.

Earlier in this section, I covered the law of balance and discussed how to calculate the number of calories needed to maintain your current weight. If your goal is to lose weight, then you need to establish a calorie deficit by reducing the number of calories you consume through food and increasing the number of calories you burn through exercise.

The best type of diet or nutrition plan will vary from person to person. Earlier, we learned about the importance of macronutrients in a healthy diet. Based on gender, height, weight, and other factors, macronutrient requirements vary. Our goals may be different, too, and the type of foods we like or can tolerate may be different.

There are so many diets out there—paleo, keto, low-carb, the list goes on—and it can be overwhelming trying to determine which diet is the best diet for you. I've experienced many failed diets in the past by following a diet that was not specific enough or aligned to my needs or goals. Which is the best diet for weight loss? My answer is: all of them work so long as there is a calorie deficit. The diet that works best for you is the diet you can stick with over the long term.

Chapter 2 Summary

◇ Energy balance is the relationship between calories consumed and the calories burned by your body through exercise and other activities. This is a very important relationship to understand.

◇ The macronutrients protein, carbohydrates, and fat play a vital role in nutrition.

◇ Micronutrients are one of the major groups of nutrients that your body needs to function properly. Micronutrients include both vitamins and minerals.

◇ Meal preparation is an effective way to prepare healthy meals and control food intake. Meal preparation is a very important skill to develop for successful weight loss.

◇ The 80/20 approach to nutrition provides more flexibility with your diet and allows you to continue eating some foods you enjoy on your free days.

◇ Improving food quality takes time and patience. The key is to choose a variety of food that you like.

◇ When it comes to your health and fitness goals, nutrition is not a "one size fits all."

◇ The diet that works best for you is the one that provides you with the best results you can stick with over the long term.

Chapter 3
Physical Pillar

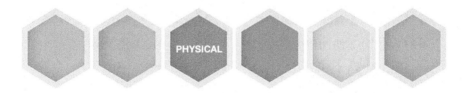

"If it doesn't challenge you, it won't change you."

- Fred DeVito

Chapter 3 Introduction

The Physical Pillar is all about your body and the importance of physical activity and exercise. The Physical Pillar will break down all the key concepts you need to know about weight training and cardio training—yes, both! Both are key for weight loss and for maintenance. In this chapter, we are going to explore the following topics:

• Body Types	• Weight-Training Exercises
• BMI	• Cardio
• Body-Fat Percentage	• Benefits of Cardio
• Major Muscle Groups	• Mode/Frequency/ Duration/Intensity
• Weight Training	• Types of Cardio
• Benefits of Weight Training	• Cardio Equipment
• Specificity/Overload/ Progression	• Steady State
• Experience Levels	• High-Intensity Interval Training (HIIT)
• Reps/Sets/Rest	• Cardio Routines

By the end of this chapter, you will have a solid understanding of weight training and cardio training, as well as the key role they both play in weight loss. This information will also help you establish an exercise routine that will support a healthy and active lifestyle. Let's jump in!

Body Types

Have you ever heard of the term "somatotypes?" "Soma" is an ancient Greek word meaning "body," and "somatotype" is a term used to describe a human body's shape and physique. The concept was originally introduced in the 1940s by William H. Sheldon, PhD, MD and later refined by other researchers over the years. Body types are based on skeletal frame characteristics and body composition.[1] There are three basic body types: ectomorph, mesomorph, and endomorph:

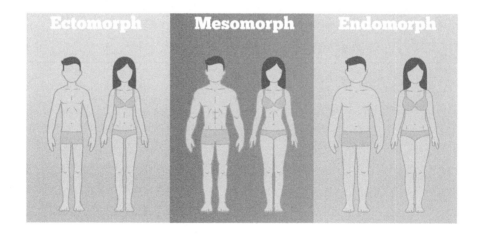

The ectomorph body type is described as typically long, slender, and thin. This body type finds it hard to gain muscle or fat mass. The mesomorph body type is described as medium build and can gain or lose weight easily. The endomorph body type is described as larger build and can gain both fat and muscle easily but struggle to lose fat. People usually are a combination of two body types, sharing characteristics from both. Understanding the different body types can provide valuable insights and help you adjust your diet and exercise plan to maximize results.

Body types have been used by experts in the health & fitness industry to design effective health & fitness plans. It's a tool to help improve lifestyle, diet, and exercise. We all respond differently to diet and exercise because our bodies come in all shapes and sizes.

Action Step

✓ Determine your body type. The website Everyday Health has a short quiz you can take to determine your body type:

https://www.everydayhealth.com/fitness/do-you-know-your-body-type/

BMI

Body Mass Index (BMI) is a measurement used to determine your level of body fat based on your height and weight. The output shows whether you are underweight, normal weight, overweight, or obese. BMI is useful because it can be used as a tool to help you gauge risk for certain lifestyle diseases.

It's important to have your BMI checked regularly. The equation for BMI is weight in kilograms divided by height in meters squared. There are charts and calculators that make it easy to find your BMI. Below is an example of a BMI chart:[2]

		Body Mass Index Table																																	
	Normal						Overweight				Obese											Extreme Obesity															
BMI	19	20	21	22	23	24	25	26	27	28	29	30	31	32	33	34	35	36	37	38	39	40	41	42	43	44	45	46	47	48	49	50	51	52	53	54
Height (inches)															Body Weight (pounds)																					
58	91	96	100	105	110	115	119	124	129	134	138	143	148	153	158	162	167	172	177	181	186	191	196	201	205	210	215	220	224	229	234	239	244	248	253	258
59	94	99	104	109	114	119	124	128	133	138	143	148	153	158	163	168	173	178	183	188	193	198	203	208	212	217	222	227	232	237	242	247	252	257	262	267
60	97	102	107	112	118	123	128	133	138	143	148	153	158	163	168	174	179	184	189	194	199	204	209	215	220	225	230	235	240	245	250	255	261	266	271	276
61	100	106	111	116	122	127	132	137	143	148	153	158	164	169	174	180	185	190	195	201	206	211	217	222	227	232	238	243	248	254	259	264	269	275	280	285
62	104	109	115	120	126	131	136	142	147	153	158	164	169	175	180	186	191	196	202	207	213	218	224	229	235	240	246	251	256	262	267	273	278	284	289	295
63	107	113	118	124	130	135	141	146	152	158	163	169	175	180	186	191	197	203	208	214	220	225	231	237	242	248	254	259	265	270	278	282	287	293	299	304
64	110	116	122	128	134	140	145	151	157	163	169	174	180	186	192	197	204	209	215	221	227	232	238	244	250	256	262	267	273	279	285	291	296	302	308	314
65	114	120	126	132	138	144	150	156	162	168	174	180	186	192	198	204	210	216	222	228	234	240	246	252	258	264	270	276	282	288	294	300	306	312	318	324
66	118	124	130	136	142	148	155	161	167	173	179	186	192	198	204	210	216	223	229	235	241	247	253	260	266	272	278	284	291	297	303	309	315	322	328	334
67	121	127	134	140	146	153	159	166	172	178	185	191	198	204	211	217	223	230	236	242	249	255	261	268	274	280	287	293	299	306	312	319	325	331	338	344
68	125	131	138	144	151	158	164	171	177	184	190	197	203	210	216	223	230	236	243	249	256	262	269	276	282	289	295	302	308	315	322	328	335	341	348	354
69	128	135	142	149	155	162	169	176	182	189	196	203	209	216	223	230	236	243	250	257	263	270	277	284	291	297	304	311	318	324	331	338	345	351	358	365
70	132	139	146	153	160	167	174	181	188	195	202	209	216	222	229	236	243	250	257	264	271	278	285	292	299	306	313	320	327	334	341	348	355	362	369	376
71	136	143	150	157	165	172	179	186	193	200	208	215	222	229	236	243	250	257	265	272	279	286	293	301	308	315	322	329	338	343	351	358	365	372	379	386
72	140	147	154	162	169	177	184	191	199	206	213	221	228	235	242	250	258	265	272	279	287	294	302	309	316	324	331	338	346	353	361	368	375	383	390	397
73	144	151	159	166	174	182	189	197	204	212	219	227	235	242	250	257	265	272	280	288	295	302	310	318	325	333	340	348	355	363	371	378	386	393	401	408
74	148	155	163	171	179	186	194	202	210	218	225	233	241	249	256	264	272	280	287	295	303	311	319	326	334	342	350	358	365	373	381	389	396	404	412	420
75	152	160	168	176	184	192	200	208	216	224	232	240	248	256	264	272	279	287	295	303	311	319	327	335	343	351	359	367	375	383	391	399	407	415	423	431
76	156	164	172	180	189	197	205	213	221	230	238	246	254	263	271	279	287	295	304	312	320	328	336	344	353	361	369	377	385	394	402	410	418	426	435	443

Source: Adapted from Clinical Guidelines on the Identification, Evaluation, and Treatment of Overweight and Obesity in Adults: The Evidence Report.

https://www.nhlbi.nih.gov/health/educational/lose_wt/BMI/bmi_tbl2.htm

I was first introduced to BMI when I was 18 years old. In the introduction to this book, I wrote about the visit I made to the doctor because my mother was very concerned about my weight and severe snoring. The doctor shared a pamphlet with me that broke down some of the basic concepts of weight management and weight loss. One item referenced in the pamphlet was a BMI chart. The chart had height listed on the left side and weight running across the top. The intersection of your height and weight provided a numerical value that represented your BMI. I was over 300 pounds, which meant I fell within the obese range on the BMI chart. An individual with a BMI of 30 or greater is considered obese. I was at a 43 BMI, which put me in the higher range of the obese category.

Getting down to a "normal weight" range seemed impossible back then. After the visit with the doctor, I set an initial goal to get down to the "overweight" range on the BMI scale. Hey, you gotta start somewhere!

Reflection

Do you know your BMI? If not, take a moment and calculate your BMI or use the chart above. You will need your current height and weight. Based on your number, what category do you fall under?

Website Link to BMI Chart: https://www.nhlbi.nih.gov/health/educational/lose_wt/BMI/bmi_tbl2.htm

Body-Fat Percentage

Measuring body-fat percentage is a useful way to assess and monitor your weight and your overall body composition. Body-fat percentage differs from BMI because it considers body composition. Knowing your body-fat percentage along with your total weight will allow you to break down your body composition: body fat versus lean mass. Lean mass is the non-fat components of your body (muscles, bones, organs, water, tendons, ligaments etc.). Lean mass is calculated by taking total body weight minus fat weight. Body-fat percentage is calculated by taking fat weight divided by total body weight and multiplying by 100.

Knowing your body-fat percentage is key to weight loss. When you think about weight loss from an overall body composition standpoint, it's the body fat you really want to target. Body fat includes essential body fat and stored body fat. Essential body fat is required for normal bodily functions and maintaining life. Stored body fat is made of excess adipose tissue that the body stores.

Body-fat percentage is used as an indicator for health. Higher levels of body fat are associated with greater risks of obesity and related lifestyle diseases. Body-fat recommendations depend on many factors, including age and gender. Below is a chart that provides the recommended body-fat percentage for both men and women by age group.

Recommended Percent Body Fat (based on American College of Sports Medicine guidelines):[3]

Age	20-29	30-39	40-49	50-59	60+
Female	16-24%	17-25%	19-28%	22-31%	22-33%
Male	7-17%	12-21%	14-23%	16-24%	17-25%

There are many ways to measure body-fat percentage. Some common methods include:

Skinfold - A caliper is used to measure the thickness of fat at one or more sites on the body.

Bioelectrical Impedance - A very small amount of electric current is passed through the body, which allows the electrical resistance of your body to be measured. Body-fat scales and handheld body-fat devices use this method.

Underwater weighing - The difference between your weight in and out of water is analyzed to determine body composition.

DEXA or dual energy X-ray absorptiometry - This is an X-ray technology that measures fat tissue.

The most accessible and practical methods I've used are skinfold tests using calipers and body-fat scales/handheld analyzers. I prefer the skinfold test because it's the least expensive and easy to perform. Skinfold tests can be done by a personal trainer at a local gym or you can purchase a set online for home use. Bottom line, keeping track of your body-fat percentage over time can provide good insights on weight-loss progress.

Action Step

✓ Determine your current body-fat percentage. If you have a body-fat scale at home, you can use it to get a snapshot. If you do not have a scale, I recommend purchasing an inexpensive skinfold caliper for home use.

Major Muscle Groups

The human body is composed of about 40 percent skeletal muscle. Skeletal muscles are the muscles that are targeted during weight training. To maximize your results with weight training, the goal should be to train all major muscle groups a minimum of two times per week. The American Heart Association recommends including moderate to high-intensity muscle-strengthening activity at least twice per week.[4] A well-rounded weight training plan will include the following major muscle groups:

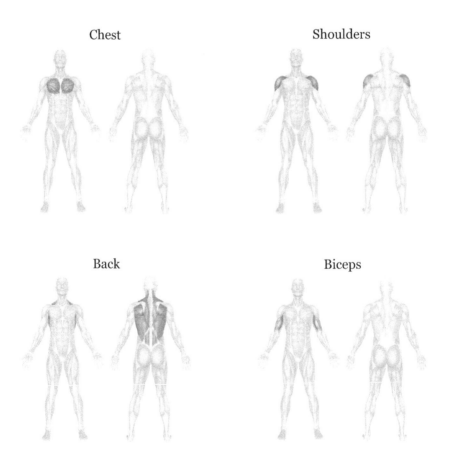

Chest

Shoulders

Back

Biceps

Triceps

Forearms

Abdominals

Glutes

Hips

Quadriceps

Hamstrings   Calves

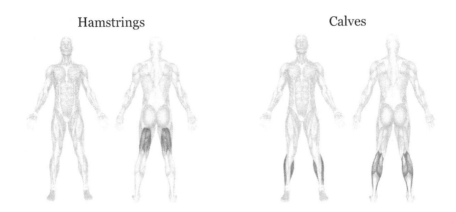

It's important to know the major muscles and how to train the muscles. Having a basic understanding of muscle anatomy is also important for preventing muscle imbalances and preventing injuries. This will provide you with basic weight-training knowledge and help you develop an overall plan to meet your goals.

I learned about the major muscle groups in college when I took a weight-training course in my senior year as an elective. I was pleasantly surprised with how much I learned about muscles and how to train them. Weight training is now a major part of my lifestyle, and I'm constantly learning and applying what I learn as a personal trainer. Now that I'm in a space where I'm helping and training others, I find it even more important to keep learning and growing this knowledge base.

Reflection

What is your favorite muscle group to train? What is your least favorite muscle group to train?

Weight Training

"Focus on the pounds you lift, not the pounds you weigh."

- Jenelle Summers

Over the years, I have developed a strong passion and respect for weight training. Weight training is a form of progressive resistance exercise. Weight training includes exercises that involve moving weights and/or body weight to strengthen muscles. If you are looking to get stronger and increase muscle size and endurance, weight training is where the magic happens. It can change the shape of your body, which will not only make you feel good but also look good.

Weight training is beneficial for both men and women. In fact, everyone who has a muscular system can benefit from weight training, including children, adults, and people with disabilities. Weight training is an efficient form of exercise to develop and maintain muscle, which is key for weight loss, as it will help increase metabolism, prevent muscle loss while losing weight, and burn more calories in the long run. Weight training has its benefits even after weight loss is achieved, as no other form of exercise can transform your body the way weight training can.

Early in my journey, I did very little weight training. My first experience with lifting weights was back when I was in high school. My brother and I had a weight bench in our room that included a cheap barbell and a few plastic plates that had sand in them. Yes, sand! We mostly used it as a clothes rack until my visit with the doctor about my weight. Shortly after that fateful visit, I began exercising by doing bench presses and jumping jacks. That's all I knew.

Over the years, my knowledge and interest grew. Now, I am a huge advocate of weight training. I am fascinated by the number of domains and methods of weight training. I'm still learning, even after many years of training. The following sections will provide everything you need to know to incorporate weight training in your weight-loss journey, from the most basic to more advanced weight-training concepts.

Reflection

Are you currently using weight training as part of your weight-loss strategy? What are some aspects of weight training where you need more information or education?

Benefits of Weight Training

If you are serious about losing weight and keeping it off, weight training is key. Weight training provides a host of benefits that are essential for weight loss and maintaining an active and healthy lifestyle.

I would like to highlight nine key benefits I found to be most impactful during my weight-loss journey, but keep in mind that this is not an exhaustive list. There are a host of other benefits.

Builds Muscle

Weight training provides stress to the muscles, which causes the muscle to break down. During the muscle repair process, it must adapt and get stronger. As muscle size increases, you will be able to lift weights more easily and for longer durations.

Boosts Metabolism

Weight training increases muscle mass, and when you increase muscle mass, your resting metabolism increases. With an increased metabolism, you will naturally burn more calories.

Great for Weight Loss and Weight Control

The best way to lose weight is a combination of a healthy diet, cardiovascular exercise (cardio), and weight training. As mentioned above, weight training increases resting metabolism, which will help you burn more calories even when you aren't working out.

Improves Balance

You need good balance to do most types of physical activity. Weight training strengthens the muscles that help you balance and keep you upright. Training muscles in the midsection of your body and legs can help improve stability and help prevent falls.

Improves Sleep

There is a strong connection between weight training and sleep. Adding weight training to your weight-loss plan will help ease any issues with insomnia and improve sleep quality. I've experienced this benefit right away when I incorporated weight training consistently. When you strengthen your muscles, your body undergoes physical changes that help overcome the stressors of training, which enable the body to produce a better quality of sleep.

Improves Self-Confidence

When weight training is performed consistently over time, you will see an improvement in how you feel and how you look. You will become more confident as you get stronger and shed the excess body fat. This improved confidence will spill over into other areas of your life.

Mind-Body Connection

Weight training requires you to know how your body functions and how exercises develop your muscles. With this knowledge, you can sculpt your body and maximize your results. As you gain more experience with weight training, you will develop a strong mind-body connection. A strong mind-body connection will allow you to increase your muscle-building potential. For example, when you increase focus on a particular muscle region during exercise, the brain will activate a greater number of muscle fibers.

Improves Cardiovascular Health

Weight training is not only good for your muscles, bones, and joints, it's also good for the heart. In fact, weight training can be just as effective as cardio for protecting the heart. A study in the March 2019 *Medicine & Science in Sports & Exercise* evaluated the exercise habits of approximately 13,000 adults who did not have cardiovascular disease. The researchers found that those who did at least one hour of weight training per week had a 40 percent to 70 percent lower risk of heart attack or stroke compared with those who did not exercise.[5]

Relieves Stress

Certain types of physical activity reduce stress by releasing endorphins. Endorphins are chemicals released by the brain during times of pain and stress. Endorphins help to improve mood and decrease stress. With the right intensity and duration, weight training can increase endorphin production.

Reflection

Which of these benefits are you most intrigued by?

Specificity/Overload/Progression

There are three key principles that define how you progress in a weight-training program. The three principles are specificity, overload, and progression.

Specificity is built around the concept of exercising the specific muscle you want to develop. For example, if you want to develop shoulders, you must focus on exercises that target shoulders. In addition, specificity also considers the goal you have for developing that muscle. Do you want to build strength, increase muscle size, or improve muscle endurance? Your goal will determine the type of program you follow.

The next principle is overload. When weight training, the muscle must be overloaded (or forced to work harder than usual) in order to stimulate change. This principle is key because, over time, muscles will adapt to training or exercise. There are several ways to apply the overload principle in +a weight-training program. Below are some of the common approaches:

- Increasing the weight
- Increasing the number of reps
- Increasing the number of sets
- Changing the rest intervals
- Changing the order of exercises

The third principle is progression. It is directly tied to the overload principle. As mentioned above, the muscles will adapt to training. Once the muscles have adapted, plateaus can occur, and the muscles will no longer be forced to work harder than normal. That means you will stop growing, gaining muscles, and getting the intended benefits of the workout. To overcome this, muscles need to be progressively overloaded. The progression in workload must be enough to stimulate improvement and keep you going in the right direction.

Mastering these principles allowed me to work out smarter and avoid some of the most common weight training pitfalls. The best way to master the principles is with consistent practice and continuous improvement. Weight training plays a huge role in weight loss and plays an even bigger role in helping to keep the weight off.

<u>Reflection</u>

In the past, have your weight-training program included any of the elements? If so, which of the three elements did the program include?

Experience Levels

Weight-training experience levels help determine the best course of action and program to follow. It's not an exact science, but it will help to make sure you are training at an appropriate frequency and intensity. The main factors that differentiate the various levels are time spent training, the type of program a person is involved in, the type of exercises involved, and the level of consistency.

Beginner

Beginning level is six months or fewer of consistent weight training. Strength gains and muscle growth happen in this stage as your muscles learn to adapt to the new demand. At this level, you are training one to three days per week, hitting all major muscle groups one to two times per week.

Intermediate

Intermediate level is one to two years of consistent weight training. At the intermediate level, strength gains and muscle growth will continue. This is based on having a specific plan and applying the weight-training principles; specificity, overload, and progression. At this level, you are training four to five days per week, hitting all major muscle groups at least two times per week.

Advanced

Advanced level is two or more years of consistent weight training. At this level, you are training at least five to six days per week and have a more advanced goal beyond weight loss or weight maintenance. This is where you see some people get into formal bodybuilding, powerlifting, or Olympic-style programs.

Below are some examples of weight training plans based on level. This is my "go to" when working with my friends, family, and coaching clients. Everyone has a different starting point and experience level.

Beginner

- 1-Day Full Body - Hit all major muscle groups one day per week
- 2-Day Full Body - Hit all major muscle groups two days per week
- (See appendix for sample Full Body weight training routine)

Beginner/Intermediate

- 3-Day Full Body - Hit all major muscle groups three days per week
- 3-Day Upper Body/Lower Body/ Full Body - Hit all major muscle groups two to three days per week. Non-consecutive days (ex. Monday, Wednesday, Friday or Tuesday, Thursday, Saturday)
- 3-Day Upper Body/Lower Body - Hit all major muscle groups two to three times per week. Non-consecutive days (ex. Monday, Wednesday, Friday or Tuesday, Thursday, Saturday)

Intermediate

- 4-Day Upper Body/Lower Body Split - Hit all major muscle groups two days per week.
- 4-Day Push/Pull/Lower Body/Upper Body - Hit all major muscle groups two days per week. One day focused on push exercises, and one day focused on pull exercises.
- (See appendix for sample upper-body and lower-body weight-training routine)

Advanced

- 5-Day Legs/Push/Pull/Lower Body/Upper Body - Hit all major muscle groups two to three times per week
- 6-Day Legs/Push/Pull/Lower Body/Upper Body - Hit all major muscle groups two to three times per week
- (See appendix for sample push and pull weight-training routine)

Consistency is key with weight training. It will maximize your weight loss and help you burn more fat. Once you lose the weight, weight training will help keep you lean and fit.

When I started weight training almost 20 years ago, I started as a beginner and especially struggled with consistency. I didn't know any better. However, I stuck with it! I eventually progressed to intermediate and then to advanced levels of weight training. It's been a fun journey applying all the knowledge I've gained over the years and helping others incorporate weight training into their weight-loss plans.

<u>Reflection</u>

What is your current weight-training level? How will this information help you with consistency and staying on track with your plan?

Reps/Sets/Rest

A common question I get is, "How many reps should I perform for each exercise?" This is a question of intensity. Let's talk about reps, sets, and rest intervals. Having a good game plan for your session will allow you to focus on what's important and not waste valuable time.

A repetition (or rep) is a single individual action of the muscles responsible for creating a movement at a joint or series of joints. Each rep involves a lengthening (eccentric) phase when you lower the weight and a shortening (concentric) phase when you lift or curl the weight. For example, a single bicep curl is one rep, or a single deadlift is one rep. The lighter the weight, the more reps you will perform. The heavier the weight, the fewer reps you will perform.

The number of reps you perform during your workout will depend on the goals you are trying to achieve. Lower reps are ideal for increasing strength. Higher reps are ideal for improving muscle endurance, and moderate reps are ideal for building muscle size. Below is a breakdown of recommended rep ranges based on training goals:[5]

Training Goals and Rep Range

Strength	1-6 Reps
Muscle Size/Definition	8-12 Reps
Muscle Endurance	15 or more Reps

Sets are a series of repetitions performed sequentially. For example, 8-12 reps of a bicep curl are a set. Many weight-training programs will have exercises falling within one to five sets. Your goals and experience level will play a key factor. Research suggests that beginners can benefit from as little as one set per exercise. Individuals with more experience or those who have specific goals can benefit from more sets per exercise.

A rest interval is the time spent resting in between sets that allows the muscle to recover. For the average weightlifter, rest periods are typically between 30 seconds and two minutes. Some advanced weight-training programs designed for maximum strength and powerlifting have rest intervals as high as five minutes. If you allow too much rest between sets you run the risk of having your muscles cool down and you may need to do a warm-up. In addition, you may also end up having a longer session if the rest intervals are too long. Below are rest-interval guidelines based on training goals:

Strength	2-5 Minutes
Muscle Size/Definition	60-90 Seconds
Muscle Endurance	30-60 Seconds

Weight training is very demanding and places stress on the body. Muscles need about 48-72 hours to fully recover between weight-training sessions. Adequate rest between sets and rest between training sessions are important for muscle recovery and development.

Action Step

✓ Determine your training goal. Are you looking to increase strength, increase muscle size or definition, or improve muscle condition?

Weight-Training Exercises

One thing I love about weight training is that you can perform it anywhere. If you don't have any equipment like dumbbells, barbells, kettlebells, or machines, you can use the best weight of all: your body weight. Weight-training exercises can be performed at home, at work, in the gym, or outside.

In this section, I provide a list of weight-training exercises grouped by major body parts, including many that do not require any additional machinery or equipment other than your body. These are exercises I have incorporated into my training program over time and exercises I have included in programs I've designed for others. This is not an exhaustive list, but rather a list of some of my favorite "go-to" exercises that helped me lose weight and build muscle.

(Note: Exercises with an asterisk* are body weight exercises)

Chest

- Push-ups*
- Incline Push-ups*
- Decline Push-ups*
- Dumbbell Chest Press
- Incline Dumbbell Chest Press
- Decline Dumbbell Chest Press
- Dumbbell Flys
- Incline Dumbbell Flys
- Decline Dumbbell Flys
- Kettlebell Chest Press
- Barbell Bench Press

- Incline Barbell Bench Press
- Decline Barbell Bench Press
- Machine Chest Press
- Machine Flys
- Cable Crossover

Shoulders

- Dumbbell Shoulder Press
- Dumbbell Front Raises
- Dumbbell Lateral Raises
- Dumbbell Upright Rows
- Dumbbell Reverse Flys
- Dumbbell Shoulder Shrugs
- Barbell Shoulder Press
- Barbell Front Raise
- Barbell Upright Rows
- Barbell Shoulder Shrugs
- Plate Front Raises
- Plate Lateral Raises
- Plate Shoulder Shrugs
- Kettlebell Front Raises
- Kettlebell Shoulder Shrugs
- Kettlebell Lateral Raises
- Machine Shoulder Press
- Machine Lateral Raises
- Machine Reverse Flys
- Medicine Ball Shoulder Press
- Medicine Ball Front Raises

Back

- Pull-ups*
- Chin-ups*
- Dumbbell Bent-Over Rows
- Dumbbell Pull-Overs
- Dumbbell Single-Arm Rows
- Barbell Bent-Over Rows
- Barbell Pull-Overs
- Kettlebell Rows
- Machine Seated Rows
- Machine Lat Pull-Downs
- Cable Seated Rows
- Cable Lat Pull-Downs
- Band Rows
- Inverted Rows

Biceps/Forearms

- Dumbbell Curls
- Dumbbell Hammer Curls
- Dumbbell Preacher Curls
- Dumbbell Concentration Curls
- Dumbbell Reverse Curls
- Seated Dumbbell Curls
- Seated Incline Dumbbell Curls
- Seated Hammer Curls
- Machine Curls
- Barbell Curls
- Barbell Preacher Curls
- Kettlebell Curls

- Cable Curls
- Cable Hammer Curls
- Band Curls

Triceps

- Diamond Push-ups*
- Dumbbell Triceps Extensions
- Dumbbell Single-Arm Triceps Extensions
- Dumbbell Triceps Kickbacks
- Dumbbell Skull Crushers
- Barbell Triceps Extensions
- Barbell Skull Crushers
- Narrow Grip Barbell Press
- Bench/Chair Dips
- Parallel Bar Dips
- Floor Dips*
- Cable Triceps Pull-Downs
- Machine Triceps Extensions
- Machine Dips
- Band Triceps Pull-Downs

Abs/Core

- Crunches*
- Sit-ups*
- Coffin Sit-ups*
- Bicycle Crunches*
- V-ups*
- Leg Raises*
- Medicine Ball Sit-ups

- Crunches on Exercise Ball
- Hanging Leg Raises
- Hanging Knee Raises
- Machine Crunches
- Side Bends*
- Dumbbell Side Bends
- Flutter Kicks*
- Scissor Kicks*
- Ankle Biters*
- High Plank*
- Low Plank*
- Side Plank*

Quads

- Bodyweight Squats*
- Forward Lunges*
- Reverse Lunges*
- Dumbbell Squats
- Barbell Squats
- Medicine Ball Squats
- Dumbbell Goblet Squats
- Barbell Front Squat
- Band Squats
- Machine Squats
- Machine Leg Press

Hamstrings/Hips/Glutes

- Romanian Deadlifts
- Dumbbell Deadlifts

- Barbell Deadlifts
- Kettlebell Swings
- Machine Seated Leg Curls
- Machine Lying Leg Curls
- Kettlebell Swings
- Hip Thrust*
- Barbell Hip Thrust
- Dumbbell Hip Thrust
- Plate Hip Thrust
- Glute Bridge*

Calves

- Bodyweight Calf Raises*
- Dumbbell Calf Raises
- Dumbbell Seated Calf Raises
- Barbell Calf Raises
- Kettlebell Calf Raises
- Machine Calf Raises
- Machine Seated Calf Raises
- Single-Leg Calf Raises*
- Dumbbell Single-Leg Calf Raises
- Medicine Ball Calf Raises

This list will serve as a great reference to assist you with designing your weight-training program. There are many options for each body part and enough variety to allow you to keep progressing. If you are on a budget or prefer to work out at home with minimal equipment, there are plenty of exercises you can do with just your body weight. The main thing is to stay active and have fun!

Action Step

✓ Review the list of exercises and take note of any exercises you are currently doing or have done in the past.

✓ Take note of any exercises you are curious about or would like to try.

Cardio

Oh yeah, you know we must talk about cardio. People tend to either love or hate cardio. I, for one, love cardio and feel it is a key component of living an active and healthy lifestyle.

Cardiovascular training, or "Cardio," refers to rhythmic exercises that raise your heart rate and breathing with the purpose of developing cardiovascular fitness. Cardio exercises usually involve large muscle groups (chest, back, quads, hamstrings, glutes, biceps, triceps, etc.) and are performed for a specified amount of time.

When performed consistently, cardio improves the function of your heart and lungs. Cardio helps your heart and lungs function better both during exercise and at rest. Cardio training plays a key role in everyday life and performance and can help achieve your weight-loss goals. Earlier, I covered the law of calorie balance and how this law applies to weight loss. Cardio training is an effective method for burning calories and helping to increase the "calories out" side of the equation.

Cardio training was very instrumental in my weight-loss journey. The key for me was to find exercises I enjoyed doing. My "go-to" cardio exercises are running, walking, cycling, and jumping jacks. I find these to be the most enjoyable, and they always leave me feeling great afterward. When I'm working with clients or helping someone with a workout plan, my number one recommendation for selecting cardio exercises is to choose exercises you enjoy doing. Keep it fun, exciting, and challenging! Remember, this is all about living an active and healthy lifestyle. It's hard to build good habits and commit to something you do not enjoy doing.

Reflection

How about you? Do you love or hate cardio?

If you love cardio, reflect on what you enjoy most about cardio.

If you hate cardio, reflect on why cardio is not enjoyable to you.

Benefits of Cardio

The benefits of cardio go beyond strengthening your heart and lungs. Cardio has a positive effect on your whole body and well-being. Below I list some of the major benefits of cardio training. Again, this is not an exhaustive list, but should be enough to spark some interest:

Great for Weight Loss

Cardio training is great for those who are looking to lose weight because it helps to burn fat and reduce calories. When you add cardio to your nutrition and weight-training regimen, you will have a killer combination for burning fat.

Improves Endurance & Physical Performance

Engaging in regular cardio training will help improve your endurance, stamina, and overall performance. This comes in handy while navigating through everyday life. Everything from playing with your kids and carrying groceries to taking a flight of stairs will be made easier with cardio training.

Improves Mood & Mental Health

Staying active can help boost your mood and mental health. Cardio training releases endorphins, which make you feel good afterward; a single session is enough to give you a boost. There are many studies that provide evidence on how exercise can reduce symptoms related to depression. According to a study found in *The International Journal of Psychiatry in Medicine,* "exercise compares favorably to antidepressant medications as a first-line treatment for mild to moderate depression and has also been shown to improve depressive symptoms when used as an adjunct to medications."[7]

Over time, cardio training can improve your self-esteem and confidence. When you get into the routine of doing cardio, you will start to feel better about yourself and become a better you.

Helps the Immune System

Cardio training can help your immune system combat certain infections you may be vulnerable to. Regular cardio training enhances your body's ability to use antibodies and white blood cells to effectively defend against potential illnesses.

Reduce Risk of Serious Disease

Cardio training reduces the risk of heart attack, high cholesterol, high blood pressure, diabetes, and some forms of cancers.

Improves Sleep

Cardio training can help improve sleep. Sleep quality and sleep duration have been shown to improve when cardio training is performed consistently. A group of researchers conducted a 12-week study to evaluate exercise training on sleep disorders. After 12 weeks of exercise, the researchers found that moderate improvements in sleep quality occurred following the exercise training.[8]

Live Longer

Many studies suggest that people who regularly perform cardio exercise will live longer than those who don't exercise on a regular basis. In addition, they may also have a lower risk of dying from causes like heart disease and certain types of cancer. For example, according to a meta-analysis that reviewed 13 different studies, eight of the studies provided evidence that regular physical activity is associated with an increase of life expectancy by 0.4 to 6.9 years.[9]

These are some great benefits. It's great to see that the benefits go well beyond weight loss and help sustain a healthy lifestyle. When I'm working with someone who is unsure about including cardio in their weight-loss plan, I focus on explaining the benefits. If you are looking for a "why," these benefits will certainly help.

Reflection

Which of the benefits listed intrigue you the most? Are these benefits enough to have cardio be a key component of your weight-loss journey?

Mode/Frequency/Duration/Intensity

Before we dive deeper into cardio training, I would like to cover some key terms. Like the concepts we covered with strength training, cardio training also requires proper progression and variation to realize its full benefits. The key variables to consider when laying out a cardio plan are mode, frequency, duration, and intensity.

Mode

Mode refers to the type of exercise. There are a lot of exercises to choose from. In the next section, I provide a list of cardio exercises. When choosing an exercise, it's important to choose exercises you enjoy and can perform safely and consistently.

Frequency

Frequency refers to how often an exercise is performed, usually recorded as the number of workouts or sessions per day or per week.

Duration

Duration refers to how long you engage in a single session of exercise. The recommended duration for beginners is 10-15 minutes. As fitness levels improve, duration can be increased based on goals.

Intensity

The intensity of your workout refers to how hard your body is working during the exercise. During cardio training, you can measure intensity using heart rate and perceived rate of exertion. The most effective methods of measuring your heart rate are to use a heart rate monitor or to count your pulse. Exercise intensity needs to be in between 60-90 percent of maximal heart rate in order to achieve ideal cardiovascular fitness levels. Maximal heart rate is estimated by subtracting your age from 220.

A good cardio-training plan requires a balance between mode, frequency, duration, and intensity. Now that we have some of the key terms covered, let's jump into some of the exercises.

Reflection

Determine your maximum heart rate by subtracting your current age from 220.

Types of Cardio

When I first started my fitness journey over 20 years ago, the only cardio I was familiar with and willing to perform was jumping jacks. Yes, old school, gym-class style jumping jacks. Back then, I wasn't aware of the variety and vast number of cardio exercises available. I've learned a lot since then and have incorporated many types of cardio exercises into my routine, such as running, cycling, boxing, etc. I still throw in some jumping jacks now and then to mix things up.

Below are different types of cardio exercises:

- Brisk Walking
- Jogging/Running
- Biking/Cycling
- Swimming
- Water Aerobics
- Kayaking
- Dancing
- Hiking
- Boxing/Kickboxing
- Martial Arts
- Rowing
- Roller Skating/Roller Blading
- Golfing
- Basketball
- Soccer
- Baseball
- Volleyball
- Racquetball

- Burpees
- Jump Rope
- Squat Jumps
- Bear Crawls
- High Knees
- Trampoline
- Hula-Hooping
- Jumping Jacks (You know I had to throw that one in there)

As you can see, there is a wide spectrum of cardio exercises. It's important to choose exercises you can perform safely and enjoy doing. If you dread working out or keep putting it off because you don't like the exercises, you will struggle to maintain consistency and meet your goals. Consistency is key! You are much more likely to stick with a routine if it's something you enjoy.

Be open to trying new exercises and experimenting. You never know what you might like until you try it. I'm glad I did. Otherwise, I'd probably still be doing only jumping jacks for my cardio.

Action Steps

✓ Review the list of cardio exercises and choose three to five cardio exercises that you would like to try.

Cardio Equipment

There are various types of cardio equipment available to help you stay active and reach your goals. You can find most of this equipment at your local gym, or you can make an investment and purchase your favorite equipment for home use. Below is a list of common cardio equipment:

- Treadmills
- Stationary Bikes
- Spin Bikes
- Air Bikes
- Recumbent Bikes
- Rowing Machines
- Elliptical Trainers
- Arc Trainers
- Stair Climbers
- Vertical Climbers
- SkiErgs

I've experimented with all the equipment listed. Some I enjoy more than others, but they all serve their purpose in providing a good cardio workout. My "go to" or favorite cardio equipment is the treadmill and stationary bike.

Safety is a top priority when using cardio equipment. When you want to try new equipment at the gym, be sure to ask a trainer or staff member to show you how to use it properly. If you bought equipment for home use, be sure to read the manufacturer's user manual and make sure that the equipment is assembled properly. Whether at home or at the gym, wear the appropriate clothing and footwear for the exercise. Lastly, respect your physical limitations. Use equipment that matches your ability and adjust the equipment for your size. I had to learn this the hard way when I used an air bike for the first time. I hopped on the bike without adjusting it and banged the crap out of my knee. If you keep these tips in mind, you will have a safe and enjoyable experience.

Reflection

What's your favorite cardio equipment? Are there any on the list you would like to try?

Steady State

Steady-state cardio is a cardio workout that is a continuous steady effort. Most cardio done over an extended period falls within the steady-state cardio training category. For example, when you see someone running for a half-hour at a steady pace, they're performing steady-state cardio.

Other categories include high-intensity interval training (HIIT), where exercises are broken down into high-intensity work/rest intervals. Many of my cardio sessions are steady-state sessions, as I do a lot of endurance training for running and cycling. We'll touch on HIIT shortly, but for now, let's focus on steady state.

Steady-state cardio is done at a consistent level of intensity, ideally a 6 out of 10 on a perceived exertion scale where 10 is an all-out max effort. Another way to measure intensity is by using heart rate. As we discussed earlier, the intensity level for steady-state cardio is roughly 60-70 percent of max heart rate. Beginners usually start out with 10-15 minutes and work up to 30+ minutes. More advanced or fit individuals often perform 60-90 minutes of steady-state cardio.

Steady-state cardio is ideal for beginners who are progressing in their fitness journey and for those recovering from injury. According to a study in the *Journal Sports Medicine Open*, low-intensity exercise results in better exercise adherence and has a lower risk of injury.[10]

Steady-state cardio burns many calories. When your goal is fat loss, 30-45 minutes at a moderate intensity is usually the sweet spot needed to get a good burn. This falls in line with the

Physical Activity Guidelines for Americans 2nd edition, which recommends adults looking to lose weight or keep it off engage in 150-300 minutes of cardio per week.[11]

<u>Reflection</u>

Are you currently performing steady-state cardio? How long are your sessions?

HIIT

While we are on the topic of cardio training, let's cover High-Intensity Interval Training, or HIIT.

HIIT takes your cardio training to another level. It is a training method that incorporates high-intensity work intervals with short, lower intensity (recovery) intervals in a single session. During the high-intensity work interval, you'll be challenging yourself almost to your max, and during the lower intensity interval, you reduce the intensity to allow for recovery. The work-to-recovery interval will vary based on the type of exercise and your current fitness level. A sample HIIT workout with a 2:1 work recovery interval might look like this: 20 seconds of sprinting followed by ten seconds of walking or 30 seconds of box jumps followed by 15 seconds of walking in place.

HIIT is a type of anaerobic training. Anaerobic means "without oxygen," and anaerobic exercises are categorized as high-intensity activities sustained over a short period of time. Since there is a lower presence of oxygen in the blood during these quick bouts of anaerobic activity, this form of exercise uses glycogen as fuel. This causes carbohydrates to break down and leave behind lactic acid. This lactic acid is what causes fatigue and discomfort after a workout. If you have ever done a full-out sprint, you know this feeling.

Recovering before the next interval is essential when performing HIIT. It forces the body to adjust between two distinct states, which provides excellent cardio conditioning. Because of the level of difficulty and intensity, HIIT workouts are usually between 10-30 minutes long. You can perform HIIT training using your body weight or with any type of cardio equipment. For example, you can use HIIT for running, rowing, indoor or outdoor cycling, jump rope, stair climbing, etc.

HIIT is an efficient way to exercise and can help you burn more calories. Several studies have shown that HIIT can elevate your metabolism for hours after exercise. For example, Tom Hazell and a team of researchers conducted a study of sprint-interval exercise and found that two minutes of sprint-interval exercise produced a 24-hour oxygen consumption similar to 30 minutes of endurance exercise.[12] This results in more calories burned after you finish exercising. If you are looking for a way to take it to the next level, HIIT may be a good option.

Steady state or HIIT?

Both types are effective and can help you reach goals. Combining steady-state and HIIT workouts is a good way to keep challenging your body and improving your overall fitness. By incorporating both training styles into your fitness routine, you'll maximize calorie burn and improve your endurance.

Reflection

Do you have any experience with HIIT workouts? If so, What is your preference, steady state or HIIT?

Cardio Routines

To wrap up the cardio section, I would like to share some of my favorite cardio routines I have picked up over the years. These cardio routines were instrumental in my weight-loss and fitness journey.

Run/Walk - Intervals

I'm a huge fan of Jeff Galloway's run/walk method. I was first introduced to this style of training when I took part in the CRIM training program years ago. My favorite run/walk intervals are 5:1, where I run for five minutes and walk for one minute. I repeat the intervals for a predetermined distance; for example, if my goal was to run three miles, I would repeat the 5:1 interval until I reached three miles.

Tabata

Tabata workouts are fun and intense. Tabata routines usually comprise eight 20-second rounds with 10-second rest breaks between each round. Each round can comprise different exercises, or you can take a pair of exercises and alternate between each round. One of my favorite Tabata routines is when I pair jump roping and shadowboxing. I jump rope for 20 seconds, take a quick 10-second break, and then shadowbox for 20 seconds. I do this for eight rounds.

Cardio Mix

As the name implies, the cardio mix is a mix of different cardio exercises done over a specific duration, with brief rest in between exercises. Because of the intensity, I usually keep these sessions to 12-15 minutes. For example, I may do a cardio mix that includes jumping jacks, high knees, shadowboxing, toe taps, windmills, mountain climbers, and jump rope. I'll perform 30 reps of each exercise with a brief rest in between for a round, then I'll set my timer for 15 minutes and perform as many rounds as I can.

Run/Bike/Run

I used to train and race in duathlons (running and biking) years ago. To train for the duathlons, I would alternate between running and biking to build up my endurance. This could be done outside using an actual road bike or indoors using a stationary bike and treadmill. For example, I would go for a two-mile run, and then hop on the bike for six miles, and then finish up with a two-mile run.

In the chapter about the Physical Pillar, you learned about your body and the importance of weight training and cardio. Moving forward, you now have all the information you need to establish an exercise routine that will help you reach your goals. You are well on your way to becoming the best version of yourself. Keep it up!

Action Steps

✓ Have you set a SMART goal for exercise? If not, take a moment to set a SMART goal for both weight training and cardio.

Chapter 3 Summary

◇ We all have different body types that respond differently to diet and exercise.

◇ Body Mass Index (BMI) is a measurement to determine body-fat levels based on your height and weight.

◇ Knowing your body-fat percentage along with your total weight will allow you to break down your body composition: body fat versus lean mass.

◇ Body measurements can provide additional insights on progress your body has made because of your weight-loss efforts.

◇ A well-rounded weight-training plan will target all the major muscle groups.

◇ There are three key principles that define how you progress in a weight-training program. The three principles are specificity, overload, and progression.

◇ Weight training provides a host of benefits that are essential for weight loss and maintaining an active & healthy lifestyle.

◇ Cardio training plays a key role in everyday life and performance. Cardio helps your heart and lungs function better both during exercise and at rest.

◇ The key variables to consider when laying out a cardio plan are mode, frequency, duration, and intensity.

◇ It's important to choose cardio exercises that you can perform safely and exercises that you enjoy doing.

Chapter 4
Social Pillar

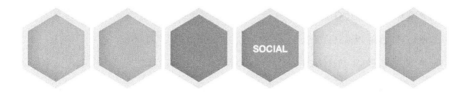

"A friend is someone who accepts your past, supports your present, and encourages your future."

- Unknown

Chapter 4 Introduction

The weight-loss journey can get lonely at times. There may be times when you feel like giving up because you may have no one to support you or hold you accountable. There may be other times where you wish there was someone there to navigate this journey with you. The Social Pillar will help fill this void.

The Social Pillar highlights key areas where you can reach out to others for support to help you along the journey. In this chapter, we will cover the following topics:

- Accountability Partners
- Friends
- Social Media
- Support Groups
- Circle of Influence
- Family
- Workout Partner
- Co-Workers

Out of all the Pillars, this is the one I had to work on the most. In the past, I tried to do everything on my own, and I found it difficult to ask others for their help. I did not see the true value of having someone support me on my journey. My perspective shifted once I was more open to seeking support from those around me. The journey became more enjoyable and fulfilling. I realized I did not have to search far to get the support I needed to meet my goals.

Accountability Partners

An accountability partner will help you tremendously when it comes to maximizing your chances of reaching your goals.

An accountability partner is someone you have established a mutual agreement with to hold each other accountable for taking action toward your respective goals. You share your goals with one another and establish a cadence to review and provide updates on progress. In addition, when you meet, you may discuss any wins, challenges, and next steps you will take to accomplish your goals. Having someone to talk to on a regular basis who will support and motivate you is huge.

This will provide you with added support and motivation, as well as any needed coaching or feedback on your progress. Accountability partners can be great sources of advice when encountering issues along the way.

I had an accountability partner during my weight-loss journey whom I checked in with on a weekly basis. I would provide updates on my progress and my plans for the coming week, and he did the same. We shared nutrition and fitness tips with one another and brainstormed ways to maximize our results.

There are many benefits to having an accountability partner. Below are some key benefits:

- Accountability partners provide added support and motivation
- They can help brainstorm or problem solve any issues you may face
- They provide you with honest feedback; both positive and constructive

- They can share ideas and strategies with you
- They provide a safe space/environment that is judgment-free

---

Action Steps

How to find the right accountability partner:

✓ Do your research and find someone that you trust and/or someone that has similar goals or has achieved similar goals. You can use social media or online forums as resources to secure a partner.

✓ Meet and set clear expectations and align on purpose and expected outcomes.

✓ Set up regular meetings and make a commitment to attend meetings. Meetings can be virtual or in person.

Friends

Friends play an important role in the Social Pillar. They can provide a huge motivational boost and can have a positive impact on your results. Having friends who support your weight-loss goals can add so much fun to the experience, as well as motivation to stay on track. Good friends may even join you for your workouts or help you plan or cook healthy meals. Friends can also be an excellent source for information like healthy recipes, trainer or coach recommendations, good gyms in the area, and so much more.

I once had a coaching client who had an amazing group of friends and social support. My client's best friend helped her with weekly meal prep and went grocery shopping with her to pick out fresh, whole food. Having this extra support from her best friend allowed her to stay on track and reach her goal weight.

I also had great support from friends during my weight-loss journey. I had a few friends who would join me on bike rides and runs. It made the experience more enjoyable, and I got better at these activities because I was able to learn and train with friends who were more experienced. I also had friends who would provide me with some healthy snacks to try out or send me recipes I could incorporate into my new, clean eating diet.

However, not all friends are good friends. In fact, some friends you should beware of! Certain friends can have a negative impact. Be on the lookout for those who do not support your goals or even unintentionally (or intentionally) sabotage your efforts. Let's face it, not all your friends will be supportive of or agree with your new lifestyle. That's OK! It's all about how you manage those relationships and how you interact with these friends. It's especially important that you share your goals and help them understand why your goals are important. If you find that this does not help or your friend still does not support your weight-loss goals, you may need to distance yourself to ensure the relationship does not cause further conflict. This way, you can stay on track and not be distracted. In addition, this may open the doors to gaining new friends or rekindling previous friendships that will have a more positive impact on your overall success.

Action Steps

✓ Reach out to a friend and invite them to a workout or healthy meal.

Social Media

Social media is where many people get their news and information on what's going on in the world. Why not use this to your advantage by following groups or individuals that can help you reach your goals? Social media can be a great tool for weight loss and can provide good quality information that will support a healthy lifestyle.

My "go-to" social media platforms are Facebook and Instagram. I currently use Facebook to share exercise and nutrition information, as well as to take part in and manage private groups or communities related to fitness and nutrition. During my weight-loss journey, I took part in various social media challenges that kept me engaged and motivated. For example, I participated in a month-long squat challenge where participants were provided with daily rep targets. Prizes were given out at the end of the challenge. It was nice to be able to meet new people who shared common goals and who wanted to provide support. This experience led me to create my own Facebook groups where I can foster an environment of support and motivation.

I also use Instagram to share information and content related to exercise and nutrition. Instagram is also a source of inspiration and motivation. This platform has introduced me to a lot of cool people from around the world who promote health and fitness. I've picked up many exercises and weight-loss tips from some of the enthusiasts and influencers I follow.

I've also gained many followers who enjoy the content I share. I try to stay consistent with my content to help others and to be a source of inspiration and motivation for those out there seeking it. Social media can be a useful tool for you, and I encourage you to leverage it to support you on your weight-loss journey.

Be on the lookout for false or misleading information on social media. When in doubt, do additional research or reach out to a trusted coach or fitness professional to validate any questionable content.

Action Steps

✓ Are you currently using any social media platforms to obtain health and fitness content? Are there any public figures or influencers you enjoy following?

Support Groups

Support groups are an excellent option for those looking for additional help with their weight-loss journey. Support groups are available in many communities, workplaces, and even online, and there are many out there that are geared toward health and fitness.

Support groups can be either formal or informal. An example of a formal support group is a workplace wellness group formed to provide support to employees looking to improve their health, while an informal support group would look like a group that naturally forms within a community and meets regularly to train together. In either case, support groups can be extremely helpful and can provide you with the support needed to keep you on track.

When joining a support group, it's important to choose a group that is positive and uplifting. The last thing you want is to join a group that has a negative atmosphere and is made up of members that are disengaged. If you find yourself in this situation, run fast and find another group.

Can't find a group? Another option is to grab some family and friends and form your own support group. Your group can be an in-person group, an online group, or both. The key to keep in mind when creating your own support group is to establish a clear purpose. By having a clear purpose, you will establish direction for the group and attract the right people.

I created an online support group using Facebook and have built a community of like-minded individuals who all want to live an active and healthy lifestyle. We share information on health, fitness, and nutrition. We also take part in various fitness challenges throughout the year. The members within the group motivate and encourage each other. Some members share success stories and others post messages on how they were inspired by other members to live an active and healthy lifestyle. This group has not only made a difference in my life and helped me reach my goals, but it has also changed the lives of so many people within the group.

Action Steps

✓ Do some research on support groups in your area. Obtain information on membership and how to join.

✓ Ask for recommendations on online support groups. Facebook has a ton of public and private groups geared toward health and fitness.

Circle of Influence

Words of wisdom can stick with you for a lifetime. I will never forget what my favorite high school math teacher told the class one day as we were preparing for a final exam. He stated, "You will end up with the same results as the five people you spend the most time with. Choose your friends wisely."

I remember thinking deeply about what my teacher said and why he said it. As I grew wiser and started experiencing life, I have come to understand how powerful influence can be.

Those closest to you—those in your closest "circle of influence"—will have the greatest influence on your life, whether you realize it or not. This holds true in all aspects, whether it's your personal, school, career, or family life. Your top five people influence your thoughts, decisions, and any actions you take. This influence can be positive and can benefit you—such as a mentor or coach you have a close relationship with. On the other hand, the influence can also be negative and even become a potential barrier. For example, you may have a close friend or relative you spend a lot of time with who lives on the wild side. Depending on where you are in life and your life goals, this relationship could cause conflicts.

You may be wondering how this applies to weight loss or living a healthy and active lifestyle. Well, some of the obstacles and challenges you will be faced with when trying to lose weight may be caused by some of the relationships and interactions with the people who are closest to you. It's a challenge living an active and healthy lifestyle when those close to you are inactive and have poor eating habits. After a while, you could find yourself back to your old habits if you do not address your circle.

Addressing your circle is easier said than done. The first step is to recognize who is in your circle of influence and determine if the relationship helps or hinders you. Once you have determined those who will help you, you will need to share your goals with them and explain why your goals are important to you. Ask for their support and let them know how they can best support you.

This approach will not work with all people in your circle. You will find that you may need to distance yourself or sever the relationship if you cannot come to terms. Choose wisely!

Reflection

Which five people do you spend the most time with?

Family

"Family is not an important thing. It's everything!"

- Michael J Fox

Family is everything! The weight-loss journey is not an easy one, but having an awesome family to support you makes all the difference. I encourage you to do everything in your power to get your family on board to support you with your goal of losing weight and living an active and healthy lifestyle.

When I speak to people who have gone through successful weight-loss transformations, I often hear about how the support of their family played a significant role in their success. I also find that their "why" is usually centered on their family and that their family is a big source of motivation to live a healthy and active lifestyle.

My family, which includes my wife, Lakisha, and my two daughters, were in my corner every step of the way. If you go back and look at my "why" that I posted earlier in the book, you will notice that several of my items were centered on my family. My family is a huge source of motivation, and I would not have achieved my goals if it were not for their unconditional love and support. They helped me stay on track and often reminded me about my goals on the days I would slip up. It was great having this support system at home.

Your family will probably be the first source you tap into in the Social Pillar. Don't hesitate to get them involved to help you with your journey. In order to get the most support from your family, they must know what your goals are and how they can best support you. Knowing is half the battle!

Action Steps

✓ Share your why and your goals with your family.

✓ Be open with them on what you need and how they can support you on your journey.

✓ Provide your family with updates on your progress and share your victories along the way.

✓ When you reach your goal, celebrate with your family!

Workout Partner

A workout partner can be a family member, friend, or co-worker who joins you on workouts regularly. This is your workout BFF or "ride or die" at the gym. If you are one of the lucky ones that have a consistent workout partner, you are truly blessed.

Good workout partners keep one another motivated and hold one another accountable. Knowing that someone is counting on you on the other end and not wanting to let them down can be just enough to get you off the couch and out the door. Having a workout partner can also make the experience much more enjoyable.

Choose a workout partner who is as dependable and committed as you are. The last thing you want is to partner up with someone who is going to drag you down or cause you to miss workouts. Remember the power of how the people who are close to you (or in your circle) can influence your outcome.

If you are not having any luck finding the right workout partner, or if your ideal workout partner is not located near you, a virtual workout partner can fill this void. Social media platforms, like Facebook and Instagram, are excellent tools to use to keep up with one another. You can create virtual gym check-ins, post-workout videos or pics, and share tips. You can also set up special challenges that you can do on a certain day or throughout the week. For example, I had a running challenge with my workout partner. The goal was to do 25 miles in one week. We pushed one another, and we both ended up completing the 25 miles. With various social media platforms and technology, you can get very creative.

Reflection

Do you currently have a workout partner? If not, is there anyone you know who would make a good workout partner?

Co-Workers

Your place of work is another source where you can gain additional support. As I mentioned previously, the journey is way more enjoyable when you enlist others to join you. Most individuals spend more waking hours in their workplace than they do at home or anywhere else. Depending on the environment you work in, you may find yourself around people who are also struggling to lose weight or looking to improve their lifestyle. Take advantage of this golden opportunity and link up with co-workers to eat a healthy lunch or to get in a group workout before clocking in for the day.

There are some significant benefits that come with teaming up with co-workers. You can find an accountability partner and/ or workout partner at work, or create a support group or office challenge to get others involved. With an office challenge, you can have periodic weigh-ins and meetings to provide support and encourage one another. As a group, you can also set goals and celebrate small wins and achievements. It's all about making progress, and it's easier (and more rewarding) to make progress together.

Many companies have implemented workplace wellness programs. If your workplace offers health or wellness services for employees, be sure to check into them. Often these services are free or included in your benefits. There may also already be support groups or committees in place that you can join to meet other employees interested in getting healthy.

During my weight-loss journey, I linked up with many of my co-workers to work out, run, and bike. I have also led and taken part in various weight-loss challenges. It was great being able to share and work toward a common goal. Through this experience, I gained some lifelong friends who enjoy staying healthy and active.

Action Steps

✓ Find out if your company or employer has a wellness program. Some companies offer many incentives and benefits to keep their workforce healthy.

Chapter 4 Summary

◇ Having an accountability partner during your weight-loss journey will provide you with added support that will help you stay motivated throughout the process.

◇ Friends can be an excellent source for information, like healthy recipes, trainer or coach recommendations, good gyms in the area, and so much more.

◇ Social media can be a great tool for weight loss. Depending on the platform, you can follow individuals, groups, influencers, or companies that provide good quality information that will support a healthy lifestyle.

◇ Support groups are available in many communities, workplaces, and online that are geared toward health and fitness.

◇ Those closest to you will have the greatest influence on your life, whether you realize it or not. This holds true in all aspects, whether it's your personal life, school, career, or family.

◇ The weight-loss journey is not an easy one, but having an awesome family to support you makes all the difference.

◇ Choose a workout partner that is dependable and committed as you are.

◇ Some of the best friendships are formed in the workplace. This is a great opportunity to link up and support one another.

Chapter 5
Spiritual Pillar

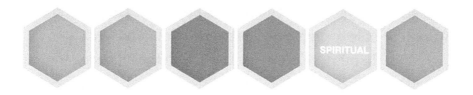

"Being spiritual has nothing to do with what you believe and everything to do with your state of consciousness."

- Eckhart Tolle

Chapter 5 Introduction

The Spiritual Pillar is all about improving your inner being and tapping into the greatness inside of you. This pillar, along with the Mental Pillar, were the biggest game changers in my health and fitness journey. I spent many years in the wilderness, lost, because I only knew part of the solution to living an active and healthy lifestyle.

You can follow the best diet and exercise plan in the world, but if your state of mind and spirit are not right, reaching your goals will be an uphill battle.

We all have an amazing power within us. We must understand ourselves and be comfortable with who we are. Once we do this, we will be able to create the best version of ourselves.

In this chapter, we are going to explore the following topics:
- Meditation
- Mindfulness
- Prayer
- Gratitude
- Love
- Happiness

These topics make up the Spiritual Pillar. When I finally fully embraced these concepts, my life improved significantly; however, you unfortunately rarely see these topics covered in the same context as weight loss. Living a healthy and active lifestyle requires a holistic approach. It's more than just diet and exercise. A healthy lifestyle includes having a healthy mind, body, and *spirit*.

After reading through each section, I want you to think and reflect on how these concepts can help you in your health and fitness journey.

Meditation

In order to change old habits and start living healthy, we must train our minds and direct our thoughts to focus on what's important in our lives. The best way to do this is through meditation.

Meditation is a practice that helps connect the mind and body to achieve a sense of calm and clarity. Meditation has been around for hundreds of years and is used by people from all around the world.

Meditation can help you gain a better understanding of yourself, including how your mind and body work. It can also help you become more in tune with your body and what you eat, making it a further useful part of your weight-loss plan. With practice, meditation can help make lasting changes to thought patterns, eating habits, and exercise habits. A 2014 study found that meditation effectively decreased binge eating and emotional eating in populations engaging in the behavior.[1]

It doesn't take much to get started. Five to 10 minutes a day of meditation is enough to reap some benefits. I started meditating during my weight-loss journey years ago and still practice meditation regularly. It is my "go-to" intervention when I need to center myself and get clarity. There are many meditation techniques out there to explore, and there are even some cool apps and guided videos online. I like the techniques that involve deep breathing or walking.

Action Steps

Here is a simple breathing technique I use regularly:

✓ Take in a deep breath through your nose

✓ Hold your breath for a few seconds

✓ Take a deep exhale through your mouth

✓ Repeat this sequence for 5-10 minutes and only focus on your breath. During meditation, it is normal for your mind to wander or for random thoughts to pop into your head. When this happens, acknowledge the thoughts, and simply return your focus to the breath.

Mindfulness

"The best way to capture moments is to pay attention. This is how we cultivate mindfulness."

-Jon Kabat-Zinn

A healthy mind leads to a healthy life, and mindfulness is a great tool that can help us achieve a healthy mind. Mindfulness teaches us the importance of being in the moment. Mindful.org describes mindfulness as "the basic human ability to be fully present, aware of where we are and what we're doing, and not overly reactive or overwhelmed by what's going on around us."[2] Mindfulness is simple, yet powerful, and with regular practice, anyone can become more mindful.

There are countless studies that support the positive benefits of mindfulness on health and weight loss. For example, researchers from McGill University found that interventions based on mindfulness proved "moderately effective for weight loss" and "largely effective" for reducing obesity-related behaviors.[3] Obesity-related behaviors include poor nutrition, overeating, physical inactivity, etc.

Learning mindfulness techniques can aid in weight loss. One of those techniques is mindful eating. Mindful eating requires you to pay more attention to food choices, hunger levels, cravings, and how your body feels before, during, and after eating. I've had great experiences with mindfulness and mindful eating. The practice has allowed me to get better at assessing my hunger levels and cravings and made me realize that if I am not careful or paying attention to what I eat, I can easily risk overeating. I've also learned to eat more slowly. I used to eat extremely fast, like there was no tomorrow. Through mindful eating, I can savor each bite and better judge when I am full. These strategies not only helped during my weight-loss journey but they are also carried over to other aspects of my life by helping me to become more aware of what's going on in my mind and body and savor the moment as it is happening.

Many studies agree that mindful eating helps you lose weight by changing your behaviors and reducing stress. Mindful eating can reduce overeating habits that directly relate to obesity. A study from the *Journal of Family Medicine and Community Health* examined the relationship between mindfulness and weight loss. The study provided evidence to support that greater weight loss is associated with increased mindfulness.[4]

Action Step - Practice mindful eating:

Focus on the food you are eating by slowing down and eating more mindfully.

✓ Eliminate distractions

✓ Eat slowly

✓ Chew your food thoroughly

✓ Focus on how the food makes you feel

Prayer

Don't worry, I'm not about to write a sermon or get overly religious in this section. I just want to touch on the power of prayer and how it helped me during my weight-loss journey and in life. My hope is that, by hearing about my experience, you will find benefit in including prayer in your arsenal for weight loss.

One of my daily habits is saying a quick prayer when I wake up in the morning, followed by reading a Bible scripture. I use the Bible App and subscribe to the daily devotionals that are available. There are so many themes available and there is usually a topic available for whatever situation you are dealing with.

After praying and reading my daily devotional, I always feel wonderful afterward. I feel like I can conquer anything the day throws at me. I do this because it gets my day started right, and it helps me connect with God.

With God, all things are possible—especially losing weight and living an active and healthy lifestyle. Losing weight can sometimes be a difficult and lonely journey. The good news is that you are not alone. My prayer and daily reading of scripture serve as a reminder that I am never alone in this, and that I always have God with me as I make the necessary changes to live an active and healthy lifestyle.

Some good alternatives to prayer are journaling or a regular gratitude practice. With journaling, you can write about the good things in your life or write about your experiences and reflect on them. An example of a gratitude practice is to think about or write about five things you are grateful for.

Reflection

Is prayer a part of your life? If so, can you think of ways prayer will help you in your journey?

Gratitude

One of the most important life lessons I learned during my weight-loss journey is centered on gratitude. Gratitude is the true key to happiness.

Gratitude is an expression of appreciation for what you have or receive, whether tangible or intangible. With gratitude, you acknowledge the goodness in your life. Giving thanks can transform your life and improve your mental, physical, and spiritual health. Research shows that the more grateful a person is, the more likely he or she is to enjoy physical and mental health.[5]

Expressing gratitude regularly has many positive benefits for health. Paul Mills and a group of researchers conducted a study that provided evidence that gratitude enhances well-being and physical health. The study examined the role of gratitude in spiritual well-being in heart failure patients.[6] Below are some of the key benefits of practicing and developing gratitude:

- Improves mental health
- Improves physical health
- Increases happiness
- Improves sleep
- Improves relationships
- Reduces stress and anxiety

Here are some ways to develop gratitude on a regular basis:

Show Appreciation - When someone does a good deed for you or gives you something, always give thanks and express appreciation. You will not only make the other person feel appreciated, but this will strengthen and build trust in your relationship.

Write a thank-you note - Writing a thank-you note is a powerful gesture. Just the mere fact that you set aside the time to write someone a personal note to thank them and show appreciation is a wonderful thing.

Pray - I touched on prayer briefly in the previous section. Prayer is a wonderful way to develop gratitude. You can use prayer to give thanks for all you have or receive from others and from God.

Meditate - You can use meditation to help develop gratitude by focusing your thoughts on what you are grateful for.

Count your blessings - Giving thanks and counting all your blessings in life can help you develop gratitude. This serves as a reminder that what you have is enough and that you are enough.

The great thing about expressing gratitude is that you can start practicing right now. You don't have to wait for the perfect moment or the right conditions. Gratitude comes from your heart.

Action Steps

✓ Try at least one of the ways to develop gratitude listed and write about your experience.

Love

Love is a powerful force. You must love yourself and love the journey you are embarking on to find true success; you must fall in love with the process of becoming the best version of yourself.

You may not be happy with your current situation, or you may not be where you expected to be in life, but loving the person you are right now is extremely important. It allows you to open your heart and mind in ways that will enhance your desired outcome.

Early in my fit-life journey, I remember being down on myself and not loving the person I saw in the mirror. I was not happy with my weight or the way I felt. I had a lot of negative feelings. These feelings certainly did not help my situation, and I spent many years in this predicament before I realized something had to change, and that change had to start with me. I had to love myself, and I had to love myself enough to take the steps to change my lifestyle.

Was it easy? No, once I got clear on who and what was important to me, things changed drastically. I gradually replaced the negative thoughts and feelings I had with positive ones. My outlook on life improved, and that empowered me to take the steps needed to change my life. If you find yourself in a similar situation, I'm here to tell you that you can tap into this powerful force.

Having negative feelings toward yourself or feeling down is a part of life. We all go through it at some point. The important thing is to be self-aware and look for ways to get back on track.

Lastly, surround yourself with people that love you and care about you. God, your family, and your friends can be a wonderful source of love and support.

__Action Steps__

✓ A great place to start is by acknowledging where you are right now and forgiving yourself. Then, look at the person in the mirror and say, "I love you," and "I believe in you." Repeat this often when you are down on yourself or don't feel the love.

Happiness

Happiness is something we all strive for. It is one of the best feelings you can experience. Merriam-Webster defines happiness as "a state of well-being and contentment."[7] Breaking down the definition, well-being involves health, prosperity, and fulfillment. Contentment is all about being satisfied with your current situation. When you break it down this way, it's clear to see that happiness begins and ends with you.

I was well into my adult life before I realized happiness comes from within. Happiness is not something that can be given to you or bought. You cannot depend on someone else to bring happiness into your life. Happiness is a state of mind, and you have all the power within you to control the amount of happiness in your life. It starts with you knowing yourself and what is truly important to you. You must appreciate and show gratitude where you are now. Be thankful for all the lessons and experiences you have had, and look forward to the journey ahead.

When I reflect on my journey and experiences in life, I find it's the little things in life that bring me happiness. The fact that I am alive is enough to be joyous and happy. As I mentioned earlier, one of the first things I do when I wake up in the morning is to thank God for blessing me with another day. I can't think of a better way to start the day. Also, being able to live an active and healthy lifestyle brings me happiness. It's not the material things or money—just simple things, the things inside of me and my state of mind.

My wish is for everyone to find happiness within. The world will be a better place because of it.

Reflection

What brings you happiness in life?

Chapter 5 Summary

◊ The Spiritual Pillar is all about improving your inner being and tapping into the greatness inside of you.

◊ Meditation can help you gain a better understanding of yourself, including how your mind and body works.

◊ A healthy mind leads to a healthy life. Mindfulness is a practice that teaches us the importance of being in the moment. Mindfulness is a meditation technique. Mindfulness is simple, yet powerful, and with practice, anyone can perform it.

◊ Gratitude is an expression of appreciation for what you have or receive, whether tangible or intangible. With gratitude, you acknowledge the goodness in your life.

◊ Prayer is a wonderful way to develop gratitude.

◊ Fall in love with becoming the best version of yourself. If you are struggling with love, the best place to start is with you.

◊ Happiness is a state of mind, and you have all the power within you to control happiness in your life.

Chapter 6
Essential Pillar

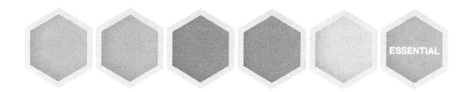

"When a flower doesn't bloom, you fix the
environment in which it grows, not the flower."

- Alexander Den Heijer

Chapter 6 Introduction

Our last Pillar is the Essential Pillar. If the Pillars were a cake, this one would be the icing. The Essential Pillar highlights additional areas that will speed up your progress and help you achieve your weight-loss goals! In this chapter, we are going to cover the following topics:

- Tracking/Monitoring Progress
- Stress Management
- Sleep
- Hydration
- Environment
- Check-ups/Physicals
- Education & Learning
- Continuous Improvement

The essentials will serve you well beyond the weight-loss phase. They will play a key part in helping you to live an active and healthy lifestyle.

Tracking/Monitoring Progress

Tracking and monitoring progress is a critical component of weight loss. This is the best way to get feedback on your plan to determine if the actions you are taking are yielding the best results. The analogy I like to use is comparing weight-loss tracking to a football scoreboard. The scoreboard provides you with the key stats and progress of the game. If you want to know the current score, check out the scoreboard. If you want to know how much time is left in the game, check the scoreboard. Need to know how many timeouts are left? Guess where you will find it: the scoreboard. Tracking for your weight-loss journey will provide you with the key stats and progress, just like the football scoreboard.

Your tracking tools can be as simple as a pen and notepad, or you can use some of the fancy mobile apps available on the market. The key is to select a method that works best for you and that you can use consistently. Trust me, tracking will serve you well in your weight-loss journey.

The equipment you'll need for tracking is a scale, tape measure, and a body-fat caliper. I recommend tracking your key stats once a week. I don't recommend daily tracking, because weight often fluctuates drastically, which can be discouraging and demoralizing to some. A weekly check-in will provide you with enough feedback on progress while reducing your exposure to the daily fluctuations.

I learned this the hard way early in my journey. I used to weigh myself daily because I did not know any better. I found myself getting angry and even quitting at times when the scale did not agree with what I thought I should be weighing.

Below are some good stats to track for your weekly weigh-ins. For weight loss, you want to see these numbers going down over time:

- Weight
- Body-fat percentage
- Waist measurement

Other stats to track if you have the tools and/or equipment:

- Blood pressure
- BMI
- Body measurements

Body Measurements

Taking measurements is another key stat to track progress for weight loss. Sometimes the scale may not provide a full picture of what's going on. There will be some weeks when the scale may not move much, or your progress may have seemed to stall. Body measurements can provide additional insights into the positive changes to your body because of your weight-loss efforts. For example, if your weight did not go down, but your waist is a half-inch smaller, that's still a win. Another example: you may have lost fat and gained muscle, resulting in the scale not changing. Taking body measurements gives you a realistic snapshot of what's happening with your body.

All you need is a body tape measure. Below are different body parts you can measure throughout your weight-loss journey to track your progress:

Chest - Measure around the torso. Place the measuring tape just under your breasts/pecs and wrap it around your back.

Bicep - Measure around the largest part of your upper arm.

Forearm - Measure around the largest part below your elbows.

Wrist - Measure around the smallest point of the wrist just below your wrist bone.

Waist - Measure around your torso starting at the navel.

Hips - Measure around the widest part at the top of the legs.

Thigh - Measure around the largest part of your upper leg.

Calves - Measure halfway between the knee and ankle.

I recommend taking body measurements once every three to four weeks. If possible, try to take your measurements at the same time of the day for consistency. Your body weight can fluctuate throughout the day. Taking measurements at the same time can reduce inconsistencies with measurements. For example, if you took your first set of measurements first thing in the morning, try to take your following measurements during the same time frame.

Food Diary

For those struggling with losing weight, a food diary—a paper or electronic diary where you keep track of the foods and meals you eat daily—is an excellent tool. Having a food diary was key to my weight-loss success. I kept track of the meals and calories I ate each day, using the MyFitnessPal app and a composition notebook. MyFitness Pal is a smartphone app and website that tracks diet and exercise. This kept me on track and made it possible for me to hold myself accountable.

The diary also served as a great learning tool because through it I could see emerging patterns and trends in my nutrition. For example, early in my journey, I noticed I was not eating enough fruit or healthy fat each week. When I noticed the trend, I took the appropriate actions to fix that problem by including more of those foods in my meals. By using the diary, I could adjust along the way to ensure I stayed on track. I still use a food diary to this day. It is a great accountability tool.

There are several food diary options for you to choose from. You can keep it simple and grab a notebook, or you can go the digital route with an app. Whichever route you decide to go, choose the method that is simple and one that you will stick with.

Action Steps

Create your personal scoreboard

✓ Determine the stats you are going to track on a weekly basis.

✓ Post your stats on your vision board.

✓ Double check to make sure the stats you are tracking have a corresponding SMART goal.

Stress Management

I flinch every time I hear the word stress. I know that there are good forms of stress, but it's not that type of stress that gets me worked up. It's the bad stress—the type of stress that could lead to serious issues if left unchecked. I feel it is important to cover stress management because chronic stress can derail your weight-loss efforts—and your life.

Stress management starts with self-awareness. I've dealt with this in the past. In my early to mid-twenties, I was under a lot of stress, and it went undetected because I did not recognize the signs. I was starting my career as an engineer, working on my master's degree, and starting my family. One important thing I learned about myself, as it relates to my relationship with food, is that I am a stress eater. When I'm stressed out, I turn to food for comfort. Unfortunately, I did not turn to healthy foods. This stress eating led to overeating, which led to excess calories that got stored as fat, which over time expanded my waistline. In addition to turning to food when stressed, I was often not very active during times of stress. This was not a good combination.

I've learned that stress was one of my triggers that would cause me to overeat. This was a key turning point in my journey. I learned about various stress management techniques, like performing regular exercise, eating healthy, getting adequate sleep, meditating, and prioritizing your workload. By learning how to manage stress, I could avoid pitfalls and triggers that would lead to bad habits.

You can manage stress and prevent weight gain associated with high levels of stress. It's all about making lifestyle changes to help you gain control of your life.

<u>Reflection</u>

Are you currently under any physical or mental stress? If yes, do you feel that your stress is impacting your ability to live an active and healthy lifestyle? Do you have an idea on what may be causing the stress? If your stress is having a major impact on your daily life, speaking with a physician or counselor may be your next best step.

Sleep

Sleep is one of the biggest essentials for successful weight loss and maintenance. I must admit, I used to think sleep was overrated. In my college days, I used to take pride in the fact that I was only getting two to three hours of sleep and still taking care of business. Little did I know, I was setting myself up for poor sleeping habits down the road. My perspective and experience with sleep have changed drastically since I was younger. I know now that sleep is vital!

Sleep rejuvenates your mind and body. When you sleep, your body heals and grows stronger. Sleep also reduces stress. A good night's sleep is restorative. You wake up with energy, ready to tackle the day. I find myself to be in a much better mood after getting a good night's sleep, no matter what the day ahead may bring.

On the other hand, sleep deprivation can have serious impacts on your health, can derail your weight-loss efforts, and can negatively impact your performance in all areas of life. Your thinking is not as sharp and you tend to not make the best decisions when you are sleep deprived, especially when making decisions about food. Sleep deprivation can lead to poor nutrition and food cravings.

The best thing you can do for yourself is to establish a sleep ritual, a habit of preparing for a good night's sleep every evening. I shared my evening routine in the habits section of the Mental Pillar chapter. Once I established a set sleep and wake time, I noticed a drastic change in my sleep quality. I now wake up feeling well-rested and ready to start my day. I also fall asleep much easier at night. Establishing a sleep ritual was one of the best things I've done to improve my sleep.

Reflection

How many hours of sleep are you getting each night? How is your sleep quality? Do you feel rejuvenated or energized in the morning when you wake up, or are you tired?

Hydration

Water plays a key role in everyday life. Drinking enough water and staying hydrated is essential for living an active and healthy lifestyle. Our bodies are made up of over 60 percent water; we need water in order to function properly, as we use water to help regulate body temperature and other bodily functions.

Proper hydration reduces fatigue and prevents you from becoming dehydrated. Dehydration occurs when your body loses more water than it takes in. When this occurs, it's difficult for your body to carry out basic functions and can have adverse effects on your health. Key takeaway: drink more water!

A good rule of thumb is to drink between 64–128 ounces of water per day. Active or larger people should be on the higher end of the range. The more active you are, the more water you need to optimize your performance. Hydration is key, before, during, and after exercise.

Earlier in the book, I provided a glimpse of my morning routine. I drink two cups of water first thing in the morning when I wake up because the body needs water after sleeping. The body loses a considerable amount of water during sleep, so it's important to replenish the lost fluids in the morning and get the day started right.

Below are 10 reasons to drink more water:
- carries nutrients and oxygen to cells
- regulates body temperature
- keeps your skin looking good
- aids in weight loss
- aids in digestion

- maintains the balance of fluid
- protects your joints and cartilage
- may prevent headache
- flushes out waste products

This is an impressive list. There are plenty of benefits to drinking water. During my weight-loss journey, I was religious about drinking enough water every day. Water is life! Below, I leave you some tips on increasing water intake. Drink up, my friend!

Action Steps - Tips to increase water intake:

✓ Drink water first thing when you wake up

✓ Drink water when you feel thirsty

✓ Drink water with every meal

✓ Drink water before, during, and after working out

✓ Replace other caloric beverages with water; for example, replace soda or juice with water.

✓ Keep a case of water in your trunk or at your place of work

Environment

Your environment plays a key role in weight loss and weight management. Where you live, work, and play influence your daily habits and routine. If your environment is filled with distractions or temptation, you will have a hard time trying to reach your goals. You want to create an environment for success.

It all begins with awareness. Are there things in your environment that can set you back or reinforce bad habits? If so, you'll want to take the steps to remove these things from your environment. You want your environment to work for you, not against you.

The best place to start is your kitchen. Start by removing all junk food and high-calorie processed food. Replace this food with healthy snacks and wholesome foods, like fruits and vegetables. Make sure the healthy snacks and foods are visible and easily accessible. If it's out of sight, it's out of mind.

Other places to assess and improve are your bedroom, workout area if you have one, your workplace, and your office or home office. Wherever you spend a significant amount of time each day, you'll want to assess and change the environment to help you reach your goals. For example, you can place your workout clothes and gym bag in a location where you can see it. This will provide you with a mental trigger and help you get into the habit of planning. Prep these items the night before so you are ready to go when the time comes to work out.

Reflection

Does your environment need some attention? Scan and assess. Do you notice any potential distractions or potential triggers? If so, take action and get your environment in order.

Check-Ups/Physicals

When was the last time you paid your doctor a visit? Visiting your doctor regularly is a must. Your doctor is one of the most important members of your personal weight-loss team. Prior to starting any nutrition program or exercise regimen, visit your doctor to make sure you are healthy and clear to begin. Once you get the green light from your doctor, it's on!

Regular check-ups allow you to mitigate any health-related issues and detect any health-related conditions. You do not want to wing it or make the wrong assumptions.

Your doctor can provide you with information and things to look out for based on your age and key health risks. Be open with your doctor and let him or her know about any health issues or concerns you have. Regular check-ups are a great way to prioritize your health and reduce the risks of chronic diseases.

A check-up or physical typically includes a health history review, physical examination, and/or lab exam. Check-ups and physicals are typically annual, but there may be instances where you need to visit your doctor more than once a year. The primary factors that determine the frequency and type of check-up include lifestyle choices, age, health condition, and family histories.

It's important to have a doctor that you feel comfortable with. I used to have a doctor back in the day who I did not enjoy going to and felt awkward speaking with about my weight. I ended up asking around for recommendations. A good friend of mine recommended my current doctor. I'm glad I made the decision to switch to them. I've now been with the same doctor for over 15 years, and I now feel comfortable speaking with my doctor about my health and any issues I'm dealing with.

Action Step

✓ Schedule a check-up or physical with your doctor or health care provider.

✓ Make a list of questions or concerns to discuss with your doctor.

Education & Learning

"When you know better you do better."

- Maya Angelou

One of the most important lessons I learned in life is that knowledge by itself is not power—*applied* knowledge is power. The day I internalized this concept was the day my life changed forever.

I love learning. A few years ago, I took the Clifton Strengths Assessment. The Clifton Strengths Assessment is an online assessment that helps discover and develop your strengths. One of my top five strengths, according to Clifton's Strength Assessment, is "learner." I'm always seeking knowledge and information and love to learn new things. When I stumble upon something that will help me in my pursuit or help me improve as a person, I find an effective way to apply this new knowledge.

Today's world is filled with a lot of educational and learning opportunities. Books, magazines, websites, blogs, social media, and both in-person and online training classes are available for you to dive deeper and gain more knowledge. Also, with mobile technology and easy-to-use mobile applications, information is literally in the palm of your hand.

Education and learning were vital during my weight-loss journey. As I mentioned earlier, I've spent a little over two decades on my journey. Over that time, I have learned lots of key lessons and gained lots of experience. I kept learning on my own and pursued formal training in nutrition, exercise, and coaching, not only to keep myself educated but also to learn how to help others who were struggling with their weight. I found that the more I learned and shared with others, the more passionate I became about helping others and making a difference.

Education and learning will also allow you to improve. We'll cover more about continuous improvement in the next topic.

Action Step

✓ Sign-up for a class or webinar on a health and fitness subject you are interested in. This will allow you to gain knowledge or insights in areas you may struggle with. There are many free resources and low-cost options available.

Continuous Improvement

I love the philosophy of continuous improvement, of the endless pursuit of incremental growth. These improvements don't happen by luck or fall out of the sky; improvements come with purposeful and intentional actions. Earlier on in my weight-loss journey, I would get complacent or remain at a certain spot after losing some weight. Old habits would creep back in, and I would have to start all over again. A continuous improvement mindset overcomes complacency and allows you to build and improve on the good habits over time.

Continuous improvement will serve you well during your weight-loss journey and will also be a key driver after you reach your goal. Reaching your weight goal is not the end; the work continues. The real goal is to maintain the active and healthy lifestyle that got you to your weight goal. Continuous improvement allows you to get better every day, mentally, physically, and spiritually, well after your goal is reached. The steps you take do not have to be monumental; the best improvements are the consistent, minor improvements that will produce significant results.

The best way to figure out the best ways to improve is through learning and practice. Keep learning about health and fitness and all the different ways you can incorporate healthy habits. You can do research online, subscribe to and read health magazines, attend a local class, or go to a seminar. The more you learn, the more you know, and the more you can do. In addition, continue practicing good habits and replacing bad habits to improve overall health and fitness. We will all get better with practice.

<u>Reflection</u>

What are some small steps you can take to improve and keep you on track?

Chapter 6 Summary

◇ Tracking and monitoring progress is a critical component of weight loss. The key is to select a method that works best for you and that you can use consistently.

◇ Stress management starts with self-awareness. Learning how to manage stress can allow you to avoid pitfalls and triggers that lead to bad habits.

◇ Sleep is one of the essentials and a key for successful weight loss and maintenance.

◇ Water plays a key role in everyday life. Drinking enough water and staying hydrated is essential for living an active and healthy lifestyle.

◇ Your environment plays a key role in weight loss and weight management. Where you live, work, and play influence your daily habits and routine.

◇ Regular check-ups allow you to mitigate any health-related issues or detect any health-related conditions. You do not want to wing it or make the wrong assumptions.

◇ One of the most important lessons I learned in life is that knowledge by itself is not power; "Applied Knowledge is Power." Education and learning will allow you to improve.

◇ We get better with practice. By practicing good habits, we improve our overall health and fitness.

Conclusion

You've made it to the end of my book! I hope you found this process to be transformative. The Fit Life Pillars are extremely effective and will help you reach your weight-loss goals. They are the same principles I followed during my life-changing transformation, and they are the principles I continue to follow in my health and fitness journey while living *That Fit Life*. These are also the same principles I use to help my clients, friends, and family members reach their health and fitness goals.

That Fit Life is like a religion to me, and I've handed my life over to it. Those who know me well can attest to this. In an earlier chapter in the book, I wrote about the importance of making a commitment. In August 2014, I made the commitment to live *That Fit Life*. Since then, everything seemed to fall into place, as I made a major transformation mentally, physically, and spiritually.

I'm on a mission to help as many people as I can to become the best version of themselves. I have a deep passion for helping people and feel that my personal experience and knowledge can really help make a difference. I hope they will make a difference for you.

Throughout the book, I provided some key action steps, reflection questions, and tips to help you apply the information immediately because I want this to be more than just informative. I want this to be an action guide for you.

Applied knowledge is power! Commit to your dreams and take action now. You have what it takes to live *That Fit Life*!

Join me on this wonderful journey!

Be more, do more! Let's go!

Acknowledgements

The first person I would like to thank is God. Through God, all things are possible.

I want to thank my beautiful wife, Lakisha Goodman, for all her love and support. You motivated me and believed in me every step of the way. I love you with all my heart.

I want to thank my wonderful daughters, Teairra and Lakeya. I do this all for them and I want to be an outstanding example and role model.

I want to thank my father, Jerry Goodman (RIH), and my mother, Velma Goodman. My mother's unconditional love and care sparked my journey.

I want to thank Self-Publising School (SPS) and my book project team for helping with the creation of my book: cover designer, editors, proofreaders, formatter, and narrator.

I also want to thank all the gym owners, trainers, runners, and coaches that I have worked with over the years.

Finally, I want to thank all my family, friends, clients, and co-workers who allowed me to help them reach their health and fitness goals. Thanks for believing in me!

About the Author

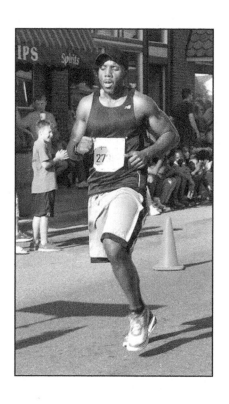

Jeremy Goodman is the Chief Fitness Officer and Owner of JGood Fitness LLC. He lives in Michigan with his wife, Lakisha, and two daughters, Teairra and Lakeya. Goodman has over 17 years of experience leading and developing high-performing teams in the utility industry and over seven years transforming lives in the health & fitness industry. He has a deep passion for health and fitness and is a Certified Health Coach, a Certified Personal Trainer, and a Certified Running Coach. He also holds a specialty certification in Fitness Nutrition. Goodman's vision is to live an active and healthy lifestyle that inspires others to do the same because he is committed to helping people reach their health and fitness goals.

Goodman started JGood Fitness LLC in 2015 to provide high-quality services and products designed to help people reach their goals and get the most out of life. JGood Fitness provides the following services and products:

- Personal Training & Small Group Training
- Online Training
- Nutrition Coaching
- Online Challenges
- Custom Running Plans
- Custom Training Plans
- Mobile App for Apple and Android
- Fitness Merchandise & Apparel

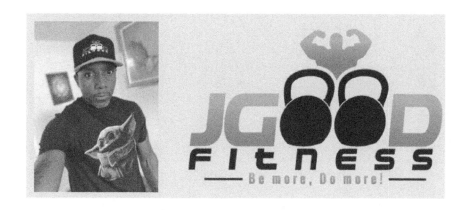

Website: https://www.jgoodfitness.com
Facebook: https://www.facebook.com/jgoodfitness
Instagram: https://www.instagram.com/jgood_fitness
Twitter: https://www.twitter.com/jgoodfitness
Snapchat: https://www.snapchat.com/add/jgood_fitness
Email: jeremy@jgoodfitness.com

90-Day Fit Life Challenge

The 90-Day Fit Life Challenge is designed to promote healthy long-term habits and to help you reach your health and fitness goals. This challenge is for all fitness levels, from beginners to fitness junkies. The challenge is for someone who wants to:

- Develop healthy nutrition and exercise habits
- Lose weight
- Improve overall fitness
- Look good and feel good
- Transform mentally, physically, and spiritually
- Get back in shape and stay in shape
- Reduce body fat
- Gain muscle
- Have more energy
- Live *That Fit Life*!

The 90 Day Fit Life Challenge is a point-based challenge. Participants get points for taking action and completing daily activities. The goal is to get as many points as possible each week. There are two ways to accumulate points in the challenge. Participants can get daily Fit Life Points and weekly Bonus Points. For more information on the challenge please visit my website:

https://jgoodfitness.com/90-day-fit-life-challenge/

References (Endnotes)

Chapter 1 – Mental Pillar

Goal Setting:

1. Covey, Stephen R. *The 7 Habits of Highly Effective People: Restoring the Character Ethic.* RosetaBooks LLC, New York, 2012

Mindset:

2. Tan, Chade-Meng. *Search Inside Yourself: The Unexpected Path to Achieving Success, Happiness (And World Peace).* Harper Collins, New York, 2012, Pages 4-5.

Habits:

3. Neal, David T., Wendy Wood, Mengju Wu, and David Kurlander. "The Pull of the Past: When Do Habits Persist Despite Conflict With Motives?" Personality and Social Psychology Bulletin 37, no. 11 (November 2011): 1428–37. https://doi.org/10.1177/0146167211419863.

Distractions:

4. "The Nielson Total Audience Report August 2020", Nielson.com, Nielson https://www.nielsen.com/us/en/insights/report/2020/the-nielsen-total-audience-report-august-2020/ Accessed 2/20/2020

5. "3-2-1: On minimalism, reading, status, and friendship" JamesClear.com https://jamesclear.com/3-2-1/january-23-2020 Accessed 2/20/2020

5Ds:

6. O'Brien, Tim. "You Can Follow the 7Ds to Success", Greensboro News & Record https://greensboro.com/you-can-follow-the-7-ds-to-success/article_45188e66-36cc-5a34-a7b4-4258df4a6d8f.html
Accessed 2/21/2020

Motivation:

7. Johnston BC, Kanters S, Bandayrel K, et al. "Comparison of Weight Loss Among Named Diet Programs in Overweight and Obese Adults: A Meta-analysis." JAMA. 2014;312(9):923–933. doi:10.1001/jama.2014.10397 Accessed 2/22/2020

8. Jack F. Hollis, Christina M. Gullion, et al. Weight Loss During the Intensive Intervention Phase of the Weight-Loss Maintenance Trial, American Journal of Preventive Medicine, Volume 35, Issue 2, 2008, Pages 118-126, https://doi.org/10.1016/j.amepre.2008.04.013.
Accessed 2/22/2020

Believe in Yourself:

9. "Self-Efficacy." *American Council on Exercise: Personal Trainer Manual* 5th Edition, American Council on Exercise, 2014

Chapter 2 – Nutrition Pillar

Calorie Requirements:

1. "Calorie" American Council on Exercise: Sports Nutrition for Health Professionals, Quincy McDonald, 2015

2. "How to Lose Weight Safely" WebMD.com, https://www.webmd.com/diet/lose-weight-fast Accessed 3/5/2020

3. "BMI Calculator" https://www.bmi-calculator.net

4. Harris, J A, and F G Benedict. "A Biometric Study of Human Basal Metabolism." *Proceedings of the National Academy of Sciences of the United States of America* vol. 4,12 (1918): 370-3. doi:10.1073/pnas.4.12.370

5. Joseph, Mini et al. "Are Predictive Equations for Estimating Resting Energy Expenditure Accurate in Asian Indian Male Weightlifters?" *Indian Journal of Endocrinology and Metabolism* vol. 21,4 (2017): 515-519. doi:10.4103/ijem.IJEM_563_16

Micronutrients:

6. "Micronutrients" World Health Organization https://www.who.int/health-topics/micronutrients#tab=tab_1 Accessed 3/7/2020

MyPlate:

7. "MyPlate" U.S. Department of Agriculture https://www.myplate.gov Accessed 3/10/2020

8. "MyPlate" U.S. Department of Agriculture Food and Nutrition Service https://www.fns.usda.gov/program/myplate Accessed 3/10/2020

Glycemic Index:

9. "Low GI Explained" Glycemic Index Foundation https://www.gisymbol.com/low-gi-explained/ Accessed 3/19/2020

Meal Quantity:

10. Bellisle, F et al. "Meal frequency and energy balance." *The British Journal of Nutrition* vol. 77 Suppl 1 (1997): S57-70. doi:10.1079/bjn19970104

Improving Food Quality:

11. "The Best Diet: Quality Counts" Harvard School of Public Health https://www.hsph.harvard.edu/nutritionsource/healthy-weight/best-diet-quality-counts/ Accessed 2/11/2021

Limit these foods:

12. Health effects of dietary risks in 195 countries, 1990–2017: a systematic analysis for the Global Burden of Disease Study 2017 https://www.thelancet.com/journals/lancet/article/PIIS0140-6736(19)30041-8/fulltext

Chapter 3 – Physical Pillar

Body Types:

1. "The 3 Somatotypes" University of Houston, Center

for Wellness Without Borders https://www.uh.edu/ fitness/comm_educators/3_somatotypesNEW.htm Accessed 1/15/2021

BMI:

2. "Calculate Your Body Mass Index" National Heart, Lung, and Blood Institute https://www.nhlbi.nih.gov/health/educational/lose_wt/BMI/bmicalc.htm Accessed 1/20/2021

Body-Fat Percentage:

3. "Body Fat Percentage" Vanderbilt University Medical Center, https://www.vumc.org/health-wellness/news-resource-articles/body-fat-percentage Accessed 1/29/2021

Major Muscle Groups:

4. "Strength and Resistance Training Exercise" American Heart Association, https://www.heart.org/en/healthy-living/fitness/fitness-basics/strength-and-resistance-training-exercise Accessed 2/1/2021

Benefits of Weight Training:

5. Liu, Yanghui, et al. *Associations of Resistance Exercise with Cardiovascular Disease Morbidity and Mortality, Medicine & Science in Sports & Exercise*: March 2019 - Volume 51 - Issue 3 - p 499-508 doi: 10.1249/MSS.0000000000001822

Reps/Sets/Rest:

6. "How to Select the Right Intensity and Repetitions for Your Clients" American Council on Exercise, https://www.acefitness.org/education-and-resources/professional/expert-articles/4922/how-to-select-the-right-intensity-and-repetitions-for-your-clients/ Accessed 2/7/2021

Benefits of Cardio:

7. Carek PJ, Laibstain SE, Carek SM. "Exercise for the Treatment of Depression and Anxiety." *The International Journal of Psychiatry in Medicine.* 2011;41(1):15-28. doi:10.2190/PM.41.1.c

8. Christopher E. Kline, PhD, E. Patrick Crowley, et al. "The Effect of Exercise Training on Obstructive Sleep Apnea and Sleep Quality: A Randomized Controlled Trial," *Sleep*, Volume 34, Issue 12, 1 December 2011, Pages 1631–1640, https://doi.org/10.5665/sleep.1422

9. Reimers, C D et al. "Does physical activity increase life expectancy? A review of the literature." *Journal of Aging Research* vol. 2012 (2012): 243958. doi:10.1155/2012/243958

Steady State:

10. Tse, A.C.Y., et al. "Effect of Low-intensity Exercise on Physical and Cognitive Health in Older Adults: a Systematic Review." *Sports Med - Open*1, 37 (2015). https://doi.org/10.1186/s40798-015-0034-8

11. "Physical Fitness Guidelines for Americans 2nd Edition," Health.Gov, https://health.gov/sites/default/files/2019-09/Physical_Activity_Guidelines_2nd_edition.pdf

HIIT:

12. Hazell, Tom J, et al. "Two minutes of sprint-interval exercise elicits 24-hr oxygen consumption similar to that of 30 min of continuous endurance exercise." *International Journal of Sport Nutrition and Exercise Metabolism* vol. 22,4 (2012): 276-83. doi:10.1123/ijsnem.22.4.276

Chapter 5 – Spiritual Pillar

Meditation:

1. Shawn N. Katterman, Brighid M. Kleinman, Megan M. Hood, Lisa M. Nackers, Joyce A. Corsica, "Mindfulness meditation as an intervention for binge eating, emotional eating, and weight loss: A systematic review," *Eating Behaviors*, Volume 15, Issue 2, 2014, Pages 197-204, https://www.sciencedirect.com/science/article/pii/S1471015314000191?via%253Dihub

Mindfulness:

2. "What is Mindfulness", Mindful.Org https://www.mindful.org/what-is-mindfulness/ Accessed 2/11/2021

3. "Mindfulness Training Shows Promise for Maintaining Weight Loss" McGill University, https://www.mcgill.ca/newsroom/channels/news/mindfulness-training-shows-promise-maintaining-weight-loss-283028

4. Dunn C, Olabode-Dada O, Whetstone L, Thomas C, Aggarwal S, et al. (2018) "Mindful Eating and Weight Loss, Results from a Randomized Trial." *J Family Med Community Health* 5(3): 1152.

Gratitude:

5. Miller, Korie D. "14 Benefits of Practicing Gratitude According to Science" Positive Pyscology.Com https://positivepsychology.com/benefits-of-gratitude/

6. Mills, Paul J et al. "The Role of Gratitude in Spiritual Well-being in Asymptomatic Heart Failure Patients." *Spirituality in clinical practice (Washington, D.C.)* vol. 2,1 (2015): 5-17. doi:10.1037/scp0000050

Happiness:

7. "Happiness." *Merriam-Webster.com Dictionary*, Merriam-Webster, https://www.merriam-webster.com/dictionary/happiness. Accessed 10/11/2021

Appendix

Sample Weight-Training Routines:

Full Body		
Exercise	Sets	Reps
Dumbbell Chest Press	3	8-12
Dumbbell Bent-Over Rows	3	8-12
Dumbbell Shoulder Press	3	8-12
Dumbbell Triceps Extension	3	8-12
Dumbbell Curls	3	8-12
Dumbbell Squat	3	8-12
Dumbbell Romanian Deadlift	3	8-12
Bodyweight Calf Raises	3	15
Crunches	3	15

Upper Body		
Exercise	Sets	Reps
Barbell Bench Press	3	8-12
Incline Dumbbell Chest Press	3	8-12
Barbell Bent-Over Rows	3	8-12
Dumbbell Pullovers	3	8-12
Dumbbell Shoulder Press	3	8-12
Dumbbell Reverse Flys	3	8-12
Dumbbell Triceps Extension	3	8-12
Dumbbell Curls	3	8-12

Lower Body		
Exercise	Sets	Reps
Barbell Squat	3	8-12
Dumbbell Goblet Squats	3	8-12
Barbell Deadlift	3	8-12
Kettlebell Swings	3	8-12
Dumbbell Calf Raises	3	8-12
Single-Leg Calf Raises	3	12-15
V-ups	3	12
High Plank	3	Hold for 45-60 seconds

Push		
Exercise	Sets	Reps
Barbell Bench Press	3-4	8-12
Incline Dumbbell Chest Press	3-4	8-12
Dumbbell Flys	3-4	8-12
Barbell Shoulder Press	3-4	8-12
Dumbbell Front Raises	3-4	8-12
Dumbbell Lateral Raises	3-4	8-12
Dumbbell Triceps Extensions	3-4	8-12
Bench Dips	3-4	15

Pull		
Exercise	Sets	Reps
Barbell Rows	3-4	8-12
Pull-ups	3-4	8-12
One-Arm Rows	3-4	8-12
Dumbbell Pullovers	3-4	8-12
Barbell Curls	3-4	8-12
Dumbbell Curls	3-4	8-12
Hammer Curls	3-4	8-12

Legs		
Exercise	Sets	Reps
Barbell Squats	3-4	8-12
Barbell Deadlifts	3-4	8-12
Leg Press	3-4	8-12
Forward Lunges	3-4	8-12
Leg Extensions	3-4	8-12
Leg Curls	3-4	8-12
Single-Leg Calf Raises	3-4	8-12

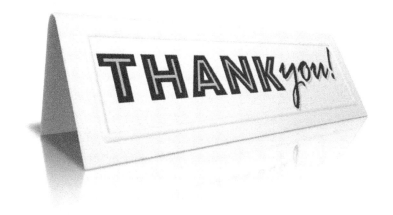

Thank You for Reading My Book!

I really appreciate all your feedback, and
I love hearing what you have to say.

I need your input to make the next version of this book and
my future books better.

Please leave me an honest review on Amazon letting me
know what you thought of the book.

Thank you very much!

Jeremy B. Goodman